Allergy Solutions

Allergies result when your immune system, incorrectly, identifies a harmless substance such as pollen as an 'intruder.' In response allergens, your body releases a family of chemicals called histamines in an attempt to rid your body of the intruder. These cause you to cough, sneeze and leak through your eyes and nose. Since the response does nothing more than cause misery, you probably want to 'turn it off.' You can with an anti-histamine such as Claritin, but there are also drug free options. So, would you rather take the drugs (side effects and all) or a natural cure for allergies (with no side effects)?

Quercetin

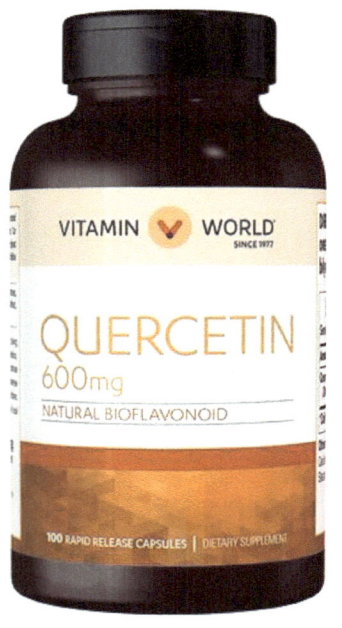

Quercetin is powerful natural cure for allergies. It blocks histamines, yet it is also provides many other health benefits including improvement of cardiovascular health, eye diseases, allergic disorders arthritis reduced cancer risk, just to name a few.[1] In addition, it naturally blocks histamines, the nasty little molecules that cause the symptoms of allergies like runny nose and sneezing.[2] Thus, you experience relief as your natural, but unmerited immune response to harmless molecules such as pollen is thwarted.

Stinging Nettle

When the body experiences any sort of 'irritation,' including from allergies, it responds by releasing various pro-inflammatory molecules. This may sound fine until you realize that inflammation results in the breakdown of tissue; that's not so good. Stinging nettle acts as a natural anti-inflammatory by inhibiting the release of these chemicals, specifically those associated with allergies.[3,4]

Oregano

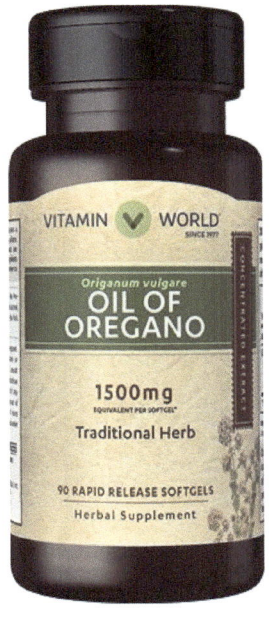

Because allergies are a reaction of your immune system , helping it out is a top priority, especially given that allergic reactions can (and in fact are supposed to) be an attempt to rid the body of a harmful intruder. Consequently, there are various forms of bacteria, viruses, funguses and other microbes floating in even the cleanest air and into our bodies all the time. Consequently, oil of oregano can kill just about all of them, plus it happens to have anti-inflammatory properties as well.[5] In short, while it is not a natural cure for allergies itself, it significantly improves your immune system, allowing it to function optimally.

References

1.   Lakhanpal P, Rai D. *Quercetin: A Versatile Flavonoid.* Internet Journal of Medical Update – EJOURNAL. 2007;2(2):22. doi:10.4314/ijmu.v2i2.39851.

2.   Weng Z, Zhang B, Asadi S et al. *Quercetin Is More Effective than Cromolyn in Blocking Human Mast Cell Cytokine Release and Inhibits Contact Dermatitis and Photosensitivity in Humans. PLoS ONE.* 2012;7(3):e33805. doi:10.1371/journal.pone.0033805.

3.   Riehemann K, Behnke B, Schulze-Osthoff K. *Plant extracts from stinging nettle (Urtica dioica), an antirheumatic remedy, inhibit the proinflammatory transcription factor NF-κB. FEBS Lett.* 1999;442(1):89-94. doi:10.1016/s0014-5793(98)01622-6.

4.   Roschek B, Fink R, McMichael M, Alberte R. *Nettle extract (Urtica dioica) affects key receptors and enzymes associated with allergic rhinitis. Phytotherapy Research.* 2009;23(7):920-926. doi:10.1002/ptr.2763.

5.   Fritz H. MA ND *Oil of Oregano | NPC. Naturopathiccurrentscom.* 2015. Available at: https://www.naturopathiccurrents.com/articles/oil-oregano. Accessed June 21, 2018.

Blood Sugar

Whenever you eat food, particularly with carbs/sugars in it, your pancreas releases a hormone called insulin. This "tells" your cells to absorb sugar. If this does not happen properly, then you end up with too much in your blood. Health problems are sure to follow. In fact, it is quite harmful in the long-run and is thought to be the reason for much of the disease we see, like diabetes, heart disease and even cancer. This is why regulating it to an overall lower blood sugar is so crucial. If (#1) your pancreas does not produce enough insulin and/or (#2) your cells do not respond properly to it, then you have diabetes.[1] Of course, there are many drugs on the market that want you to buy them. But natural blood sugar control is a far better answer than drugs!

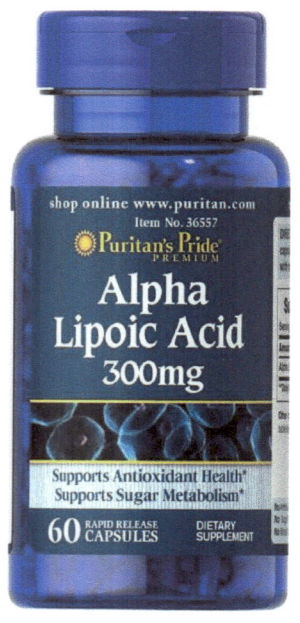

Alpha Lipoic Acid (ALA)

This amazing molecule does exist in some foods but isn't super common. It is one of the few powerful, free radical fighting antioxidants that is both fat and water soluble. Thus, it can eliminate harmful waste products anywhere in your body. Most antioxidants only work in watery or fatty parts but not both.[2] But ALA is also a great tool in the battle against diabetes because it fights problem #1 by mimicking insulin. This will automatically lower the level of sugar in your blood. So, even if your pancreas is not producing enough on its own, ALA encourages your cells to absorb insulin anyway. The result is natural blood sugar control.[3] In addition, it is effective in the treatment of diabetic neuropathy (a type of nerve damage that results from diabetes).[2]

Cinnamon

Cinnamon is a well-known herb for sugar regulation as well. Besides, it tastes good too! In particular, it is thought to tackle problem #2 by reducing insulin resistance of your cells.[4] Even with enough insulin, if your cells don't respond, you will still end up with high levels of sugar in your blood and all the nasty health outcomes associated with it. Plus, studies have proven that cinnamon is quite good at natural blood sugar control and, although unrelated, cholesterol too.[5]

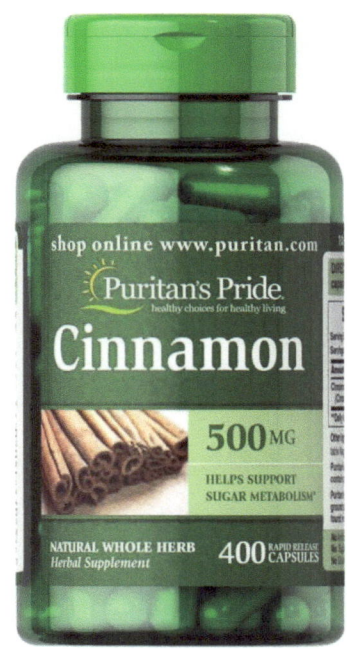

Gymnema Sylvestre

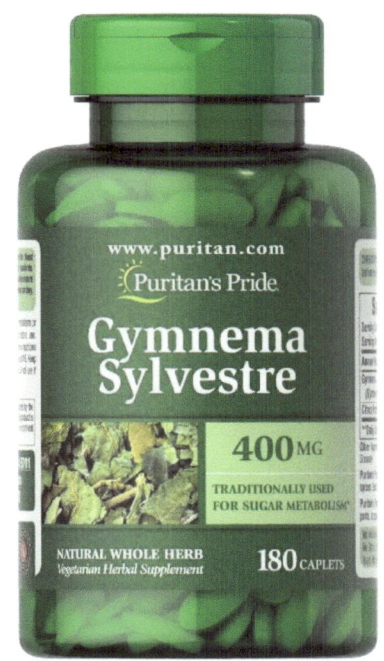

Within your pancreas are special cells known as beta cells. They have two jobs; produce insulin and release it when sugar levels start rising.[6] Oftentimes diabetes results from the destruction or otherwise malfunction of these cells because your sugar level doesn't go down like it is supposed to after a meal. However, gymnema sylverstre actually repairs these cells somehow and even promotes weight loss.[7,8] Of course you should focus on eating lower blood sugar foods (namely low carb and super low sugar) but food won't repair your beta cells!

References

1.   What is Diabetes? | NIDDK. (2018). Retrieved from https://www.niddk.nih.gov/health-information/diabetes/overview/what-is-diabetes

2.   Alpha Lipoic Acid. (2018). Retrieved from http://healthlibrary.brighamandwomens.org/library/diseasesconditions/adult/Kidney/19,AlphalipoicAcid

3.   Nahar, P., Shah, S., Kshirsagar, M., Ghongane, B., & Udupa, A. (2013). A comparative study of effects of omega-3 fatty acids, alpha lipoic acid and vitamin E in type 2 diabetes mellitus. Annals Of Medical and Health Sciences Research, 3(3), 442. doi: 10.4103/2141-9248.117954

4.   Cinnamon and Diabetes. (2018). Retrieved from https://www.webmd.com/diabetes/cinnamon-and-benefits-for-diabetes

5.   Khan, A., Safdar, M., Ali Khan, M., Khattak, K., & Anderson, R. (2003). Cinnamon Improves Glucose and Lipids of People With Type 2 Diabetes. Diabetes Care, 26(12), 3215-3218. doi: 10.2337/diacare.26.12.3215

6.   Cernea, S., & Dobreanu, M. (2013). Diabetes and beta cell function: from mechanisms to evaluation and clinical implications. Biochemia Medica, 266-280. doi: 10.11613/bm.2013.033

7.   Baskaran, K., Ahamath, B., Shanmugasundaram, K., & Shanmugasundaram, E. (1990). Antidiabetic effect of a leaf extract from Gymnema sylvestre in non-insulin-dependent diabetes mellitus patients. Journal Of Ethnopharmacology, 30(3), 295-305. doi: 10.1016/0378-8741(90)90108-6

8.   Pothuraju, R., Sharma, R., Chagalamarri, J., Jangra, S., & Kumar Kavadi, P. (2013). A systematic review of Gymnema sylvestre in obesity and diabetes management. Journal Of The Science Of Food And Agriculture, 94(5), 834-840. doi: 10.1002/jsfa.6458

Bone Strength

Building a strong bone structure is paramount, but it is easy (and common) to allow bones to slowly but surely weaken. Bone loss can be related to your genes but is usually from an inadequate diet. Since your cells need a little bit of calcium (about 1% of your total) and other minerals all the time, there always has to be a certain amount in your bloodstream. When there isn't, your body 'steals' some from your bones. When there is, your body adds to your bones.[1,2] So, you can see how this could lead to bone loss over the years and diminished bone health.

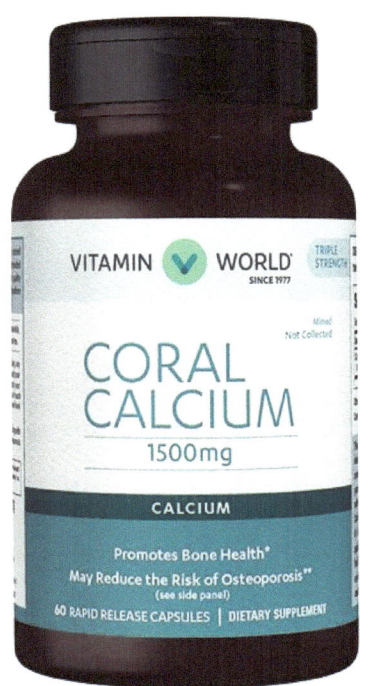

Calcium

As you might expect, calcium, although not the only mineral in bone, is by far the most abundant. Of course, other minerals are essential as well and that's where coral calcium comes in. As the name implies, it is derived from coral mined from coastal ocean areas and happens to contain a multitude of trace minerals in addition to calcium.[3] It also absorbs much better than the form of calcium you tend to find in most supplements.[4]

Magnesium

Consequently, magnesium is also a particularly important mineral for bone health, representing about 15 grams in the bones (about 1/2 lb.) while about the same amount circulates throughout the body. In fact, it participates in more than 300 enzymatic systems. A particularly important one is the formation of DNA .[3,5] This mineral is also helpful in the absorption of calcium.[6] After all, what good is it to take calcium if it doesn't absorb like it otherwise could?

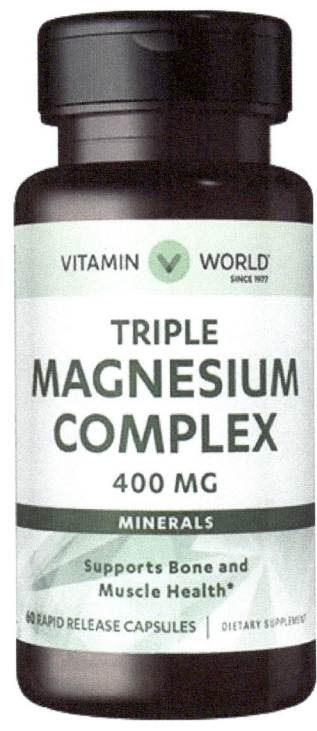

Vitamin D

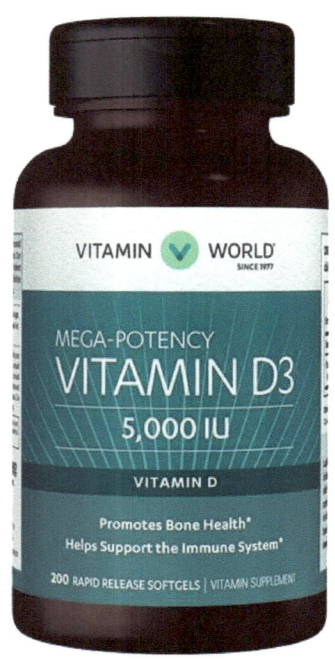

While it may be true that vitamin D is called a vitamin, it is actually more like an enzyme. When the radiation from sunlight contacts the skin, it forces a chemical in the skin to change into a useful form of vitamin D. Nevertheless, many folks are deficient in this nutrient, a huge contributor to the absorption of calcium. While it is vital for the perpetuation of a strong bone structure, it also reduces the risks of a whole slew of diseases including cancer, multiple sclerosis, autoimmune disorders, cardiovascular disease and type 1 diabetes.[7,8]

It is especially important to consume vitamin D3. Although there are three forms, not ironically called vitamin D1, vitamin D2 and vitamin D3, D1 and 2 are synthetic and far less effective. Only D3 is naturally occurring and while D1 and 2 are created in the lab and are certainly a source of vitamin D, they are not nearly as effective as the natural form.

References

1.   Wisse B, David Z. *What causes bone loss?* : MedlinePlus Medical Encyclopedia. *Medlineplusgov.* 2016. Available at: https://medlineplus.gov/ency/patientinstructions/000506.htm. Accessed June 21, 2018.

2.   *Drugs & Medications. Webmdcom.* 2018. Available at: https://www.webmd.com/drugs/2/drug-64799/coral-calcium-oral/details. Accessed June 21, 2018.

3.   Palacios C. *The Role of Nutrients in Bone Health, from A to Z. Crit Rev Food Sci Nutr.* 2007;46(8):621-628. doi:10.1080/10408390500466174.

4.   ISHITANI K, ITAKURA E, GOTO S, ESASHI T. *Calcium Absorption from the Ingestion of Coral-Derived Calcium by Humans. J Nutr Sci Vitaminol.* 1999;45(5):509-517. doi:10.3177/jnsv.45.509.

5.   *Magnesium. Odsodnihgov.* 2018. Available at: https://ods.od.nih.gov/factsheets/Magnesium-HealthProfessional/. Accessed June 21, 2018.

6.   *Nutrition's dynamic duos – Harvard Health. Harvard Health.* 2009. Available at:

https://www.health.harvard.edu/newsletter_article/Nutritions-dynamic-duos. Accessed June 21, 2018.

7.   Grant W, Holick M. *Benefits and Requirements of Vitamin D for Optimal Health: A Review. Alternative Medicine Review.* 2005;10(2):94-111. Available at:

http://anaturalhealingcenter.com/documents/Thorne/articles/vitamin_d10-2.pdf. Accessed June 21, 2018.

8.   Holick M. *Sunlight and vitamin D for bone health and prevention of autoimmune diseases, cancers, and cardiovascular disease. Am J Clin Nutr.* 2004;80(6):1678S-1688S. doi:10.1093/ajcn/80.6.1678s

Brain Health

In a very real way, you are your brain. Think about it….If you lost any other body part, you would still be you, but not if you lose your mind. Since the brain is responsible for all the feelings, thoughts and actions that make us human, it really is YOU.[1] We worry about our stomach, liver, intestines, prostate and so on, as we should, yet it is easy to neglect our brain health. Consequently, they need "food" too. But to function at their best, it is essential to provide that for them.

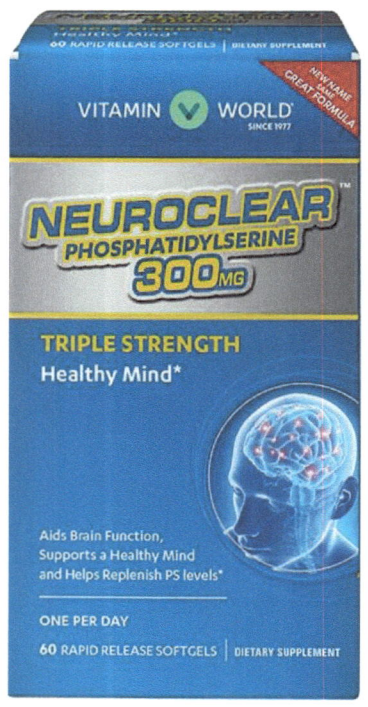

Phosphatidylserine (PS)

Every cell in your body is surrounded by a membrane composed of phospholipids (a special type of fat) and a little bit of protein, carbohydrates and cholesterol. In fact, his membrane is a lot like the front door of your home. Above all, its job is to keep good stuff in and bad stuff out. It just so happens that in your brain cells, one of these phospholipids, called phosphatidylserine (or PS), is the most common.[2] Thus, if you always have enough PS, you always ensure maximum brain health. In fact, PS supplementation has been shown to have a lot of positive effects on memory, focus and even athletic performance.[3]

Fish Oil

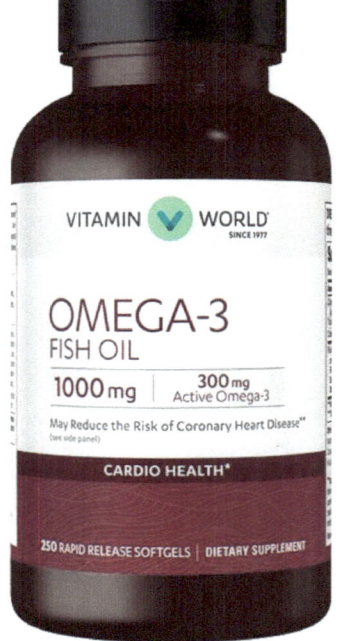

You may have already heard that fish oil is great for a lot of reasons. Well, you heard right because fish oil, among other things, has been shown to be a great supplement for improving brain function and avoiding disease.[4] In fact, the DHA in fish oil works hand in hand with phosphatidylserine to strengthen cell membranes, especially in the brain.[2] At any rate, give it what it needs, and it works better!

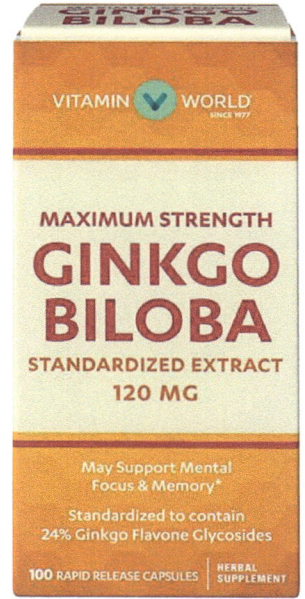

Ginkgo Biloba

Ginkgo, from one of the oldest living tree species, has been touted as a brain health enhancer for years. In brief, the benefit is thought to lie in its blood-thinning and antioxidant properties. As your blood becomes thinner, it can more easily and effectively make its way into the tiny vessels of your brain, ensuring proper oxygenation as well as free radical destruction. Studies have shown it to be both effective and ineffective, but nonetheless there are many folks who swear by it. However, be cautious if you are taking any medications as ginkgo often interacts with them. So, make sure and check.[5]

References

1.   *Brain Anatomy Core Information*. *Princetonbrainandspinecom*. 2018. Available at: https://www.princetonbrainandspine.com/brain/brain-anatomy/. Accessed June 22, 2018.

2.   Alberts B. *Molecular Biology Of The Cell*. 6th ed. New York, NY [u.a.]: Garland Science; 2015.

3.   *Phosphatidylserine*. *Uofmhealthorg*. 2015. Available at: https://www.uofmhealth.org/health-library/hn-2896001. Accessed June 22, 2018.

4.   Pearson K. *How Omega-3 Fish Oil Affects Your Brain and Mental Health*. *Healthline*. 2017. Available at: https://www.healthline.com/nutrition/omega-3-fish-oil-for-brain-health. Accessed June 22, 2018.

5.   Nordqvist J. *Health benefits of Ginkgo biloba*. *Medical News Today*. 2017. Available at: https://www.medicalnewstoday.com/articles/263105.php. Accessed June 22, 2018.

Cancer Relief

The current number of new cancer cases in the U.S. is 439.2 per 100,000 adults. More than 1/3 of all people in the U.S. will get cancer at least once in their life. In addition, we spend $147.3B per year dealing with this plague.[1] So what can you do? First of all, there is no guarantee for avoiding it, but there are many things you can do, and not do, to lower your risk. One risk reducing factor is what you put in your body. Of course you should eat a healthy diet, but there are many nutrients that can be beneficial that you will probably not get enough of from food alone.[2] The following are 3 heavy-weight cancer preventing and/or cancer fighting supplements. Of course, I can't guarantee that anything will cure you, but there is strong evidence for them to at least provide some cancer relief.

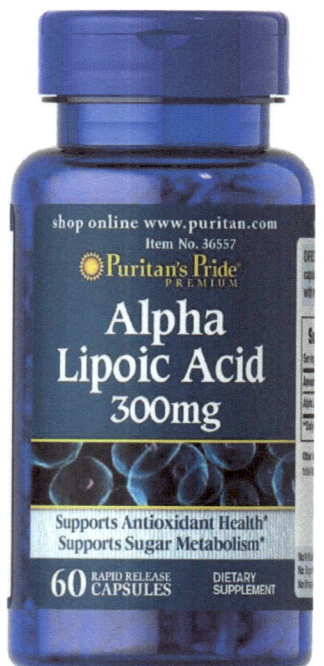

Alpha Lipoic Acid (ALA)

There are a million antioxidants out there, all of which may reduce your cancer risk. They do this by neutralizing damaging free radicals which can cause cancer and other diseases.[3] You consume some antioxidants every day, especially in fruits and vegetables, but they all differ. Some dissolve in and thus are only effective in water. Others only in fat. Thus, few antioxidants do this job in both watery AND fatty areas of your body. ALA is one of these exceptions, which makes it one of the best cancer fighting supplements. Since it neutralizes free radicals, it prevents cancer-causing damage to cells to occur in the first place. Furthermore, it has been shown to *trick* cancer cells into actually killing themselves. [4] That's sort of the definition of cancer relief!

Vitamin D

You may know vitamin D as the sunshine vitamin because your skin makes it when it comes in contact with rays from the sun. What you may not know is the widespread deficiency of vitamin D. In fact, having too little vitamin D has strong ties to colon, breast, ovarian and prostate cancer. And so, vitamin D is one of the most significant cancer fighting vitamins. Also, because vitamin D helps calcium absorb properly, a lack of this vitamin is also harmful to your bones.4 Not surprisingly, vitamin D and calcium together has been shown to reduce a woman's risk for all types of cancer.[5] In any case, vitamin D is involved in a multitude of biochemical processes in the body. Thus not having plenty in your diet can spell disaster for your health even if it doesn't result in cancer.[6]

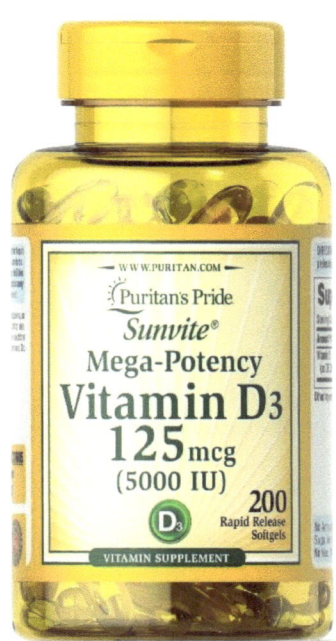

Shark Cartilage

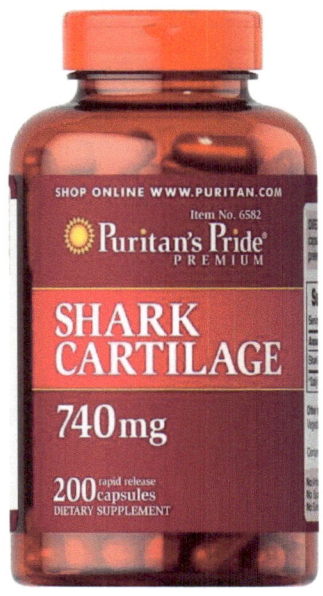

Although you don't hear about this one much anymore, it might be the best of the cancer fighting supplements out there. Since sharks don't get cancer, if you take shark cartilage, you won't either, right? In fact, some sharks do get cancer, it is just very uncommon.[7] However, it is clear that shark cartilage works as an anti-angiogenic, meaning it prevents the formation of new blood vessels.[8] Of course, cancer cells need blood, and lots of it. Shark cartilage is thus thought to prevent cancer cells from getting enough blood and therefore dying.

There is much controversy surrounding shark cartilage and so you will have to decide for yourself if it is worth taking. Some experts claim it is the Holy Grail of cancer treatment while others call it nothing more than pseudoscience.[6,8] Nevertheless, there are many survivors who attribute it to cancer relief and recovery.

References

1.   Cancer Statistics. National Cancer Institute. https://www.cancer.gov/about-cancer/understanding/statistics. Published 2019. Accessed May 16, 2019.

2.   CDC'S Second Nutrition Report: A Comprehensive Biochemical Assessment Of The Nutrition Status Of The U.S. Population. Center for Disease Control and Prevention; 2007:1-4. https://www.cdc.gov/nutritionreport/pdf/4page_%202nd%20nutrition%20report_508_032912.pdf. Accessed May 28, 2019.

3.   Novotny L, Rauko P, Cojocel C. alpha-Lipoic acid: the potential for use in cancer therapy. Neoplasma. 2008;55(2):81-6.

4.   Poprac P, Jomova K, Simunkova M, Kollar V, Rhodes CJ, Valko M. Targeting Free Radicals in Oxidative Stress-Related Human Diseases. Trends Pharmacol Sci. 2017;38(7):592-607.

5.   Lappe JM, Travers-gustafson D, Davies KM, Recker RR, Heaney RP. Vitamin D and calcium supplementation reduces cancer risk: results of a randomized trial. Am J Clin Nutr. 2007;85(6):1586-91.

6.   Holick MF. Vitamin D deficiency. N Engl J Med. 2007;357(3):266-81.

7.   Ostrander GK, Cheng KC, Wolf JC, Wolfe MJ. Shark cartilage, cancer and the growing threat of pseudoscience. Cancer Res. 2004;64(23):8485-91.

8.   Sheu JR, Fu CC, Tsai ML, Chung WJ. Effect of U-995, a potent shark cartilage-derived angiogenesis inhibitor, on anti-angiogenesis and anti-tumor activities. Anticancer Res. 1998;18(6A):4435-41.

Depression Help

Depression is no fun at all and is different than just being unhappy. You don't care about things that you once did, sleep too much or can't sleep at all, lose your appetite and so on. Genetics, personality, brain chemistry and environment are all risk factors for depression, but it is entirely treatable. In the medical field the answer is almost always drugs, but there are also natural products that can create a natural depression cure.[1]

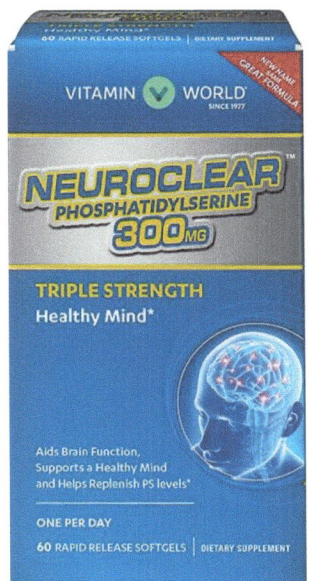

Phosphatidylserine (PS)

Every cell in your body is surrounded by a membrane composed of phospholipids (a special type of fat) and a little bit of protein, carbohydrates and cholesterol. In fact, this membrane, like the front door of your home, keeps good stuff in and bad stuff out. It just so happens that in your brain cells, one of these phospholipids, called phosphatidylserine (or PS), is much more abundant.[2] If you always have enough PS, you always ensure maximum brain function and are thus better equipped against disorders such as depression. In fact, studies have shown PS to be effective in treating a slew of brain disorders, including depression.[3]

St. John's Wort

Two common causes of depression are excessive re-uptake of serotonin and nor-epinephrine, two chemicals in the brain strongly associated with mood. Your brain cells release these neurotransmitters as a way of communicating with one another and once released, enzymes recycle them and the process begins again. Of course, this all happens in fractions of a second yet in some folks the process actually works too fast and something is needed to slow it down. Many depression drugs on the market do this such as Cymbalta (duloxetine).[4] Interestingly, St. John's Wort is a natural herb that has a similar effect, having shown to be effective in treating mild to moderate

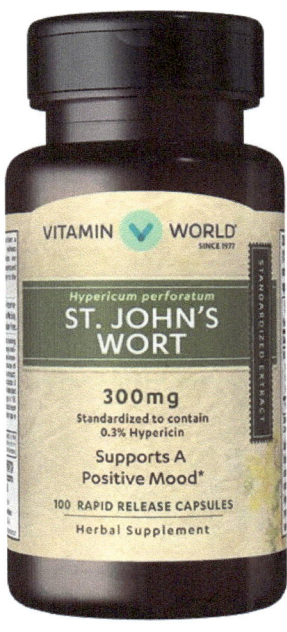

depression. Although it is a great option, it does interact with many medications, so be sure to check if you are taking any drugs.[5]

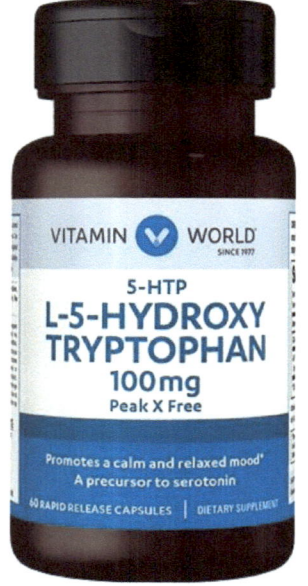

5-Hydroxytryptophan (5-HTP)

It has been understood for decades that depression results from an issue with brain chemistry, most notably neurotransmitters, serotonin being a major player. Perhaps this is why drugs are typically considered the answer rather than a natural depression cure. Nonetheless, the problem can often be the production of serotonin itself. The brain produces serotonin and does so by chemically transforming tryptophan (and amino acid) into 5-hydroxytryptophan (5HTP) and then to serotonin. However, consumption of tryptophan does not guarantee enough 5HTP, so no, eating more turkey won't do the trick. Your body still only produces a certain amount. However, the consumption of 5HTP does provide much more insurance that proper amounts of serotonin will be produced and studies have shown that supplementation of 5HTP does in fact have a positive effect on depressive symptoms as more serotonin is made.[6]

References

1.   *What Is Depression?*. Psychiatryorg. 2018. Available at: https://www.psychiatry.org/patients-families/depression/what-is-depression. Accessed June 23, 2018.

2.   Alberts B. *Molecular Biology Of The Cell. 6th ed*. New York, NY [u.a.]: Garland Science; 2015.

3.   Benton D, Donohoe R, Sillance B, Nabb S. *The Influence of Phosphatidylserine Supplementation on Mood and Heart Rate when Faced with an Acute Stressor*. Nutr Neurosci. 2001;4(3):169-178. doi:10.1080/1028415x.2001.11747360.

4.   Dugan S, Fuller M. *Duloxetine: A Dual Reuptake Inhibitor*. Annals of Pharmacotherapy. 2004;38(12):2078-2085. doi:10.1345/aph.1e084.

5.   Lawvere S, Mahoney M. *St. John's Wort*. Am Fam Physician. 2005;72(11):2249-2254. doi:10.1001/jama.284.20.2649-jbk1122-2-1.

6.   Meyers S. *Use of Neurotransmitter Precursors for Treatment of Depression*. Alternative Medicine Review. 2000;5(1):64-71. doi:10.1001/jama.282.17.1682-jbk1103-3-1.

Digestive Care

The digestion of food begins in the mouth where we chew to break food into smaller pieces as it is bathed in saliva. Once we swallow the food (or drink) enters the stomach where strong acid and digestive juices begin the chemical breakdown at the molecular level. Carbs, fats and proteins are all 'chain molecules' and only when they are broken down to individual parts can they be digested as they continue through the small intestine where most of the absorption occurs.[1] Naturally, when this process doesn't work quite right some pretty unappealing health outcomes can result. Likely, you have experienced some of them before like diarrhea and indigestion. Even worse though can be malnutrition. You might actually eat enough, but not get enough nutrients![2]

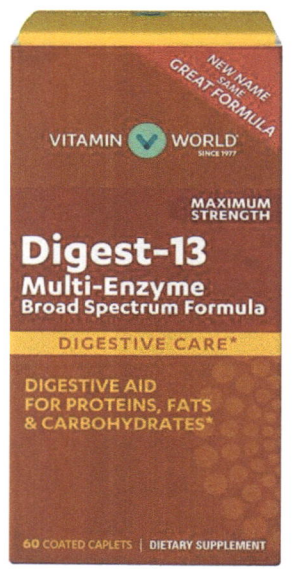

Digestive Enzymes

Digestive enzymes all fall into 3 families: proteases, lipases and amylases. Furthermore, each has the job of breaking the chemical bonds between, respectively, proteins, fats and carbs. This happens all the way through your intestines as your food slowly makes its way from your stomach to your…well, toilet. The lining of your digestive tract can only absorb food when it is broken down into its smallest "pieces," so digestive enzymes represent a crucial part of this process. When sufficient enzymes are present, your body will receive the maximum nutrition possible, but if your natural enzyme production is not at its peak (and it decreases with age among other things), food that might have made it into your body ends up in your…well, toilet.[2]

Fiber

There are actually many different fibers, but they all have one thing in common. They are carbohydrates that can't be broken down in the digestive tract but are still necessary for proper digestion. Fibers mix with food and form a sort of gel that makes its way through the stomach and intestines. Because it is a gel, it can 'reach' into small folds in the intestines and remove particles left behind that might otherwise someday might cause some problems up to and including cancer.[3]

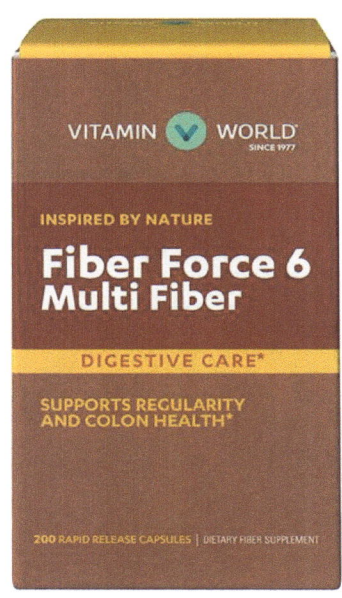

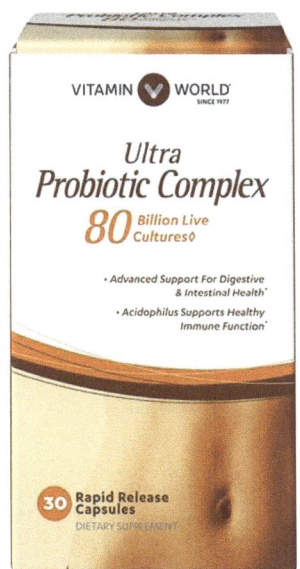

Probiotics

Acidophilus is one of the most important types of "good" bacteria in your body, but not the only one. In fact, there are 100's of types of friendly bacteria in your guts. Since they are bacteria, they are chemically 'armed to the teeth' against invaders that might normally make you sick. Unlike digestive enzymes, probiotics are living cells not unlike those throughout your body and must consume to survive, so they actually 'eat' some of the food you digest, often fibers. In fact, you can blame these guys the next time you clear a room because when they consume food particles they also release methane gas. They are regularly used to treat all sorts of digestive problems including irritable bowel syndrome, inflammatory bowel disease, inflammation of the colon, "bad" bacterial growth in the intestines, constipation, recovery from bowel surgery and so on.[4]

References

1. Medeiros D, Wildman R. *Advanced Human Nutrition. 3rd ed*. Burlington: Jones and Barlett Learning; :34-53.

2. Roland J. *Why Are Enzymes Important? Enzymes and Digestion*.
Healthline. https://www.healthline.com/health/why-are-enzymes-important. Published 2018. Accessed July 7, 2018.

3.   Staff. *How to add more fiber to your diet*. Mayo Clinic. https://www.mayoclinic.org/healthy-lifestyle/nutrition-and-healthy-eating/in-depth/fiber/art-20043983. Published 2018. Accessed July 7, 2018.

4.   *Lactobacillus: MedlinePlus Supplements*. Medlineplus.gov. https://medlineplus.gov/druginfo/natural/790.html. Published 2018. Accessed July 8, 2018.

Eye Power

It's really easy to over "look" eye health because often we only think about it when problems arise. Of course, if you already have issues, doing something about it is essential, but it is also important to keep your eyes healthy to avoid potential problems. In fact, your eyes are arguably the most complex organs, next to your brain. Thus, providing sufficient nutrients is crucial as so much can go wrong.

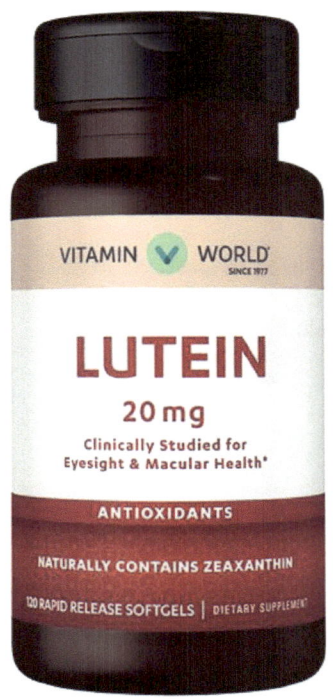

Lutein

Lutein is a very effective antioxidant. This means that it eliminates waste products naturally produced by your body before they have a chance to cause problems. Because of this, lutein can neutralize these toxins in the eyes that, over time, cause damage. Consequently, this damage eventually results in diseases like macular degeneration. The reason lutein is particularly important is that it also functions as a part of what makes up the retina and lens of the eye. So not only does it stave off damage to cells in the eye, it is an essential part of what makes up the eye itself.[1]

Bilberry

Bilberry is also another great source of antioxidants and other beneficial nutrients that can protect eye cells from damage by neutralizing free radicals that are on a constant search for cells to injure.[2] However, it also plays an important role in eye function, specifically night blindness. Although it is only legend, it is believed that during World War II, pilots accidently discovered that consuming bilberries before a night mission substantially improved their ability to see in the dark. Remember too that these guys already had great eyesight or the Air Force would have weeded them out as pilots. So, imagine how effective it could be for you! In any case, bilberry

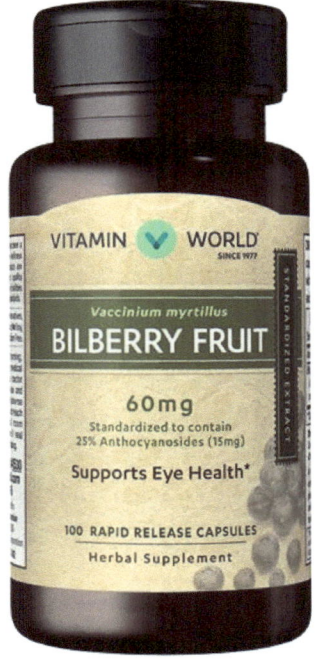

has been shown to be effective in the treatment of a multitude of eye disorders. In addition, it fights infections, kidney stones, diarrhea, cholesterol, varicose veins and atherosclerosis.[3]

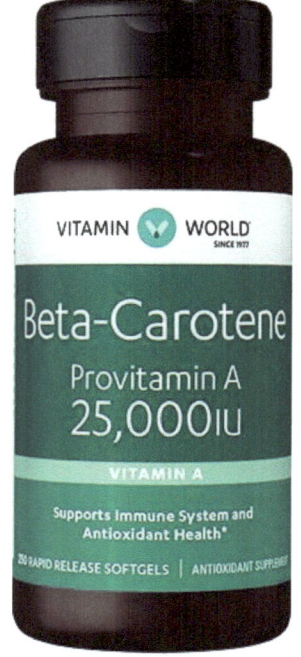

Beta Carotene

Beta carotene is a "precursor" to vitamin A. This means that it is not vitamin A, per se, but can be converted to Vitamin A as the body needs it. Vitamin A itself is fat soluble, meaning that any extra stores in fat and can potentially build up to toxic levels over time. However, excess beta carotene is not fat soluble. Instead, it is stored in the liver until it is converted to vitamin A. Thus, it cannot build to toxic levels.[4] Like lutein and bilberry, beta carotene is important for eye health and function. In fact, deficiency eventually results in the complete loss of the cornea of the eye. This is a common problem in undernourished third world populations. Egyptians even used it to treat eye problems by squeezing liver juice into patient's eyes and then feeding them the rest (liver is very high in vitamin A).[5]

References

1.   Ma L, Lin X. *Effects of lutein and zeaxanthin on aspects of eye health*. J Sci Food Agric. 2010;90(1):2-12. doi:10.1002/jsfa.3785

2.   Burdulis D, Sarkinas A, Jasutiene' I, Stackevicene' E, Janulis V. *Comparative study of anthocyanin composition, antimicrobial and antioxidant activity in bilberry (Vaccinium myrtillus L.) and blueberry (Vaccinium corymbosum L.) fruits*. Acta Pol Pharm. 2009;66(4):399-408.

3.   *Bilberry | Encyclopedia.com*. Encyclopedia.com. https://www.encyclopedia.com/sports-and-everyday-life/food-and-drink/food-and-cooking/bilberry. Published 2018. Accessed July 13, 2018.

4.   *beta-Carotene*. Pubchem.ncbi.nlm.nih.gov. https://pubchem.ncbi.nlm.nih.gov/compound/beta-carotene#section=Top. Published 2018. Accessed July 13, 2018.

5.   Maron D. *Fact or Fiction?: Carrots Improve Your Vision*. Scientific

American. https://www.scientificamerican.com/article/fact-or-fiction-carrots-improve-your-vision/. Published 2014.

Accessed July 13, 2018.

Heart Vigor

Your heart is a unique organ, different than all the others because it never rests. It speeds up as you increase activity and slows as you decrease activity and pumps more than a gallon of blood per minute,[1] but never, ever stops. When it does, you die. This is not meant to be a scare tactic, but to remind you that taking care of your heart health is very important. This is especially true if you have a heart condition or had heart problems in the past. Consequently, what you put in your body has a huge impact on how this amazing pump works for good or bad. Thus, the best heart health supplements should be part of your daily intake.

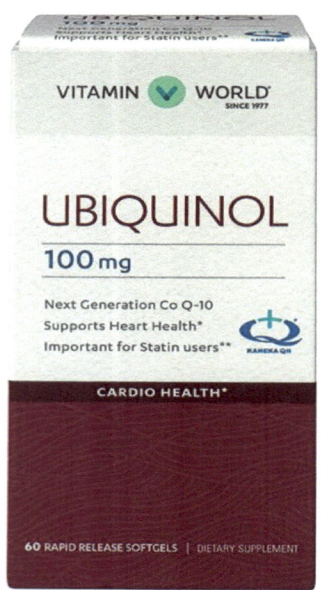

Coenzyme Q-10 / Ubiquinol

In the first place, CoQ-10 is a nutrient that helps your cells convert food into energy. This is especially important to the heart that is producing energy all the time.[2] In fact, this is why it is one of the best heart health supplements available. Consequently, it comes in two forms, ubiquinone, or CoQ-10 (the inactive form) and ubiquinol that your cells can use immediately. Your heart, especially with age, doesn't always get enough to provide optimal health.[3] As a matter of fact, it doesn't just protect the heart either, it protects all your cells from free radical damage as a powerful antioxidant.[4]

However, in a more ironic vein, statin drugs, which improve heart health by decreasing cholesterol, actually depletes this vital nutrient (remember how it is essential in the production of energy in cells of the heart?).[5] So if you are taking one of these (Lipitor, Zocor, any of the "cors"), you should doubly consider this supplement.

Fish Oil

It turns out that fish oil has about a zillion health benefits. And of course, some of those belong to your heart, which is why it is one of the great heart health supplements. Subsequently, there are two significant fats found in it, the short names for which are EPA and DHA. These both fit in the "good fats" category unlike saturated or trans-fat. In any case, fish oil has been shown to reduce triglycerides (fat in the blood).[6] It also reduces the risk of coronary heart disease, hypertension and prevents some arrhythmias (unusual heart beat).

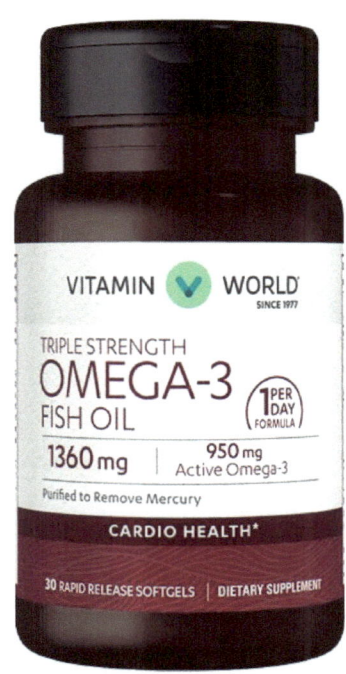

Despite the benefits, some folks worry about mercury and other toxins in fish products. While it is true that fish can be contaminated, most are within "acceptable" levels and pills are distilled, a fancy way of saying the toxins are removed.[7] This is especially true of the products you will find here.[8] Incidentally, we will not recommend a product that is anything but top-notch.

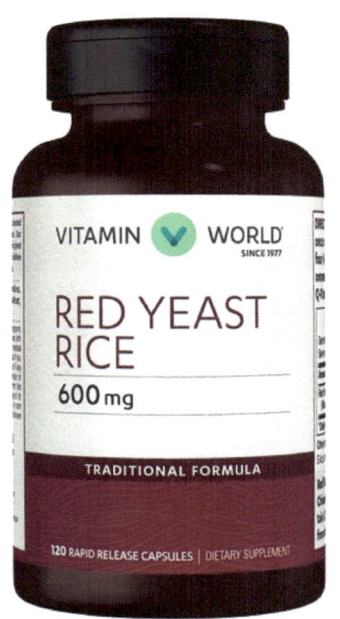

Red Yeast Rice

You have certainly heard of statin drugs like Lipitor and Zocor that lower cholesterol. In fact, you may already be taking one, but it turns out that they lower levels of CoQ10. But didn't we just say that CoQ-10 is essential to the proper function of your heart?[9] One of the common side effects of these drugs is muscle pain, likely because the muscles (including the heart) can't produce enough energy. In fact, supplemental CoQ-10 reduces pain resulting from statins significantly.[9] Red yeast rice is a statin as well, and powerful in the realm of heart health supplements, but is all natural. It is even used as an alternative to statin drugs for patients that cannot tolerate them due to their side effects. As it turns out, it works great at helping your body manage cholesterol[11] and thus greatly reduce your chances of a heart attack.

References

1.   Marieb E. *Essentials Of Human Anatomy & Physiology. 10th ed*. Boston: Benjamin Cummings; 2012:368.

2.   *CoQ10: What are the Heart Health Benefits? – Cleveland HeartLab, Inc*. Cleveland HeartLab, Inc. http://www.clevelandheartlab.com/blog/horizons-coq10-what-are-the-heart-health-benefits/. Published 2018. Accessed July 22, 2018.

3.   Ernster L, Forsmark-Andre P. *Ubiquinol: an endogenous antioxidant in aerobic organisms*. Clin Investig. 1993;71(S8). doi:10.1007/bf00226842

4.   Murphy M. *Understanding and preventing mitochondrial oxidative damage*. Biochem Soc Trans. 2016;44(5):1219-1226. doi:10.1042/bst20160108

5.   Zlatohlavek L, Vrablik M, Grauova B, Motykova E, Ceska R. *The effect of coenzyme Q10 in statin myopathy*. Neuro Endocrinol Lett. 2012;33 Suppl 2:98-101.

6.   Eslick G, Howe P, Smith C, Priest R, Bensoussan A. *Benefits of fish oil supplementation in hyperlipidemia: a systematic review and meta-analysis*. Int J Cardiol. 2009;136(1):4-16. doi:10.1016/j.ijcard.2008.03.092

7.   Sidhu K. *Health benefits and potential risks related to consumption of fish or fish oil*. Regulatory Toxicology and Pharmacology. 2003;38(3):336-344. doi:10.1016/j.yrtph.2003.07.00

8.   *Vitamin World Reviews by ConsumerLab.com with Ratings from Quality Tests*. ConsumerLab.com. https://www.consumerlab.com/Search/Vitamin-World-Review. Published 2018. Accessed November 25, 2018.

9.   Passi S, Stancato A, Aleo E, Dmitrieva A, Littarru G. *Statins lower plasma and lymphocyte ubiquinol/ubiquinone without affecting other antioxidants and PUFA*. BioFactors. 2003;18(1-4):113-124. doi:10.1002/biof.5520180213

10.   Caso G, Kelly P, McNurlan M, Lawson W. *Effect of Coenzyme Q10 on Myopathic Symptoms in Patients Treated With Statins*. Am J Cardiol. 2007;99(10):1409-1412. doi:10.1016/j.amjcard.2006.12.063

11.   Becker D. *Red Yeast Rice for Dyslipidemia in Statin-Intolerant Patients*. Ann Intern Med.

2009;150(12):830. doi:10.7326/0003-4819-150-12-200906160-00006

12.   *HDL (Good), LDL (Bad) Cholesterol and Triglycerides*.

Heart.org. http://www.heart.org/HEARTORG/Conditions/Cholesterol/HDLLDLTriglycerides/HDL-Good-LDL-

Bad-Cholesterol-and-Triglycerides_UCM_305561_Article.jsp#.W1tvtNJKi70. Published 2018. Accessed July 27,

2018.

Immune Function

Your immune system refers to your body's ability to fight infection, stay healthy and avoid sicknesses and disease. Just like an army needs weaponry to defend their country, your immune system needs the proper nutrition to defend itself from invaders that come in the form of bacteria, viruses, toxins and so forth. At every moment your immune cells are waging this battle because these potential invaders are all around us. Even in the very air we breathe! Thus, we must provide them with the building blocks they need to keep fighting a never-ending war.

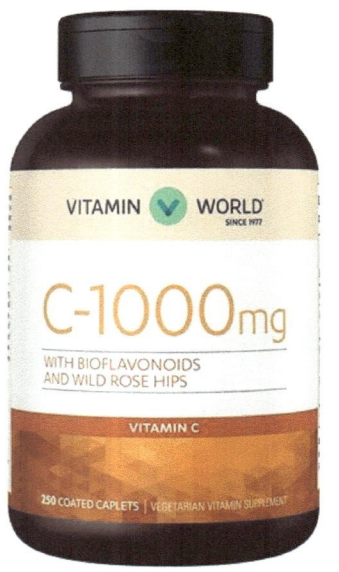

Vitamin C

Vitamin C, also called ascorbic acid, is an amazing nutrient for your immune function. Although unlike most animals, humans don't make their own. Thus, we must obtain it from food and/or supplements. Since your body cannot make collagen without it and it is also a very powerful antioxidant, which neutralizes damaging free radicals, it is invaluable to your structure as well as your health.

It is so powerful in fact that it is promoted as a means to prevent or treat numerous health conditions including cancers, heart disease, eye diseases, the common cold and even blood poisoning.[1,2] In fact, it literally kills some cancer cells outright, such as common types of colorectal cancer.[3] In addition to being such a tremendous antioxidant, it also "recharges" other antioxidants that have already been used up fighting free radicals.[1]

Echinacea

Echinacea is a flower native to North America that is commonly used in supplement form to boost immune function.[4] For many years folks have used it to prevent and treat the common cold in addition to generally boosting the immune system. The research is a bit mixed and seems to indicate that echinacea does not necessarily reduce the length of a cold, but does impact prevention.[4,5] North American Indians and eventually early settlers have used Echinacea for hundreds of years to kill germs, relieve pain, treat poisonous snake and insect bites, toothaches, sore throat, wounds and even diseases such as mumps smallpox and measles. They used it because it "works" and research has verified its ability to improve immune function.[7]

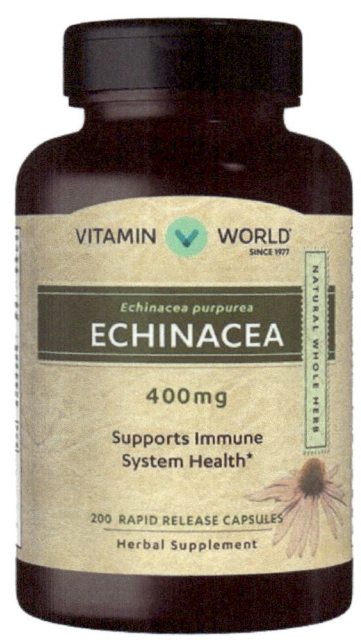

Oil of Oregano

No doubt you have had this herb in foods, but did you know how amazing it can be as an immune system aide? It is a natural anti-microbial, meaning it kills just about anything alive that may hurt you. Bacteria, viruses, fungi, worms, and even many parasites cannot withstand its effects[8] and the benefits don't stop there. That is why it is used to treat an innumerable list of conditions from acne and athlete's foot to high cholesterol and dandruff.[9] Normally your own immune system is working overtime to manage the various life-forms that are attempting to take over your body, but oil of oregano takes care of many of these intruders on its' own, freeing up your natural defenses in much the same way as antibiotics.[10]

References

1.   Office of Dietary Supplements – Vitamin C. Ods.od.nih.gov. https://ods.od.nih.gov/factsheets/VitaminC-HealthProfessional/. Published 2018. Accessed July 27, 2018.

2.   Wilson J. Mechanism of action of vitamin C in sepsis: Ascorbate modulates redox signaling in endothelium. BioFactors. 2009;35(1):5-13. doi:10.1002/biof.7

3.   Yun J, Mullarky E, Lu C et al. Vitamin C selectively kills KRAS and BRAF mutant colorectal cancer cells by targeting GAPDH. *Science*. 2015;350(6266):1391-1396. doi:10.1126/science.aaa5004

4.   Echinacea. NCCIH. https://nccih.nih.gov/health/echinacea/ataglance.htm#hed1. Published 2018. Accessed August 11, 2018.

5.   Linde K, Barrett B, Bauer R, Melchart D, Woelkart K. Echinacea for preventing and treating the common cold. *Cochrane Database of Systematic Reviews*. 2006. doi:10.1002/14651858.cd000530.pub2

6.   Ross S. Echinacea purpurea. *Holist Nurs Pract*. 2016;30(1):54-57. doi:10.1097/hnp.0000000000000130

7.   McMillen B, Mulvhill C. About Echinacea. Pitt.edu. https://www.pitt.edu/~cjm6/w98echin.html. Published 2018. Accessed August 11, 2018.

8.   Force M, Sparks W, Ronzio R. Inhibition of enteric parasites by emulsified oil of oregano in vivo. *Phytotherapy Research*. 2000;14(3):213-214. doi:10.1002/(sici)1099-1573(200005)14:3<213::aid-ptr583>3.0.co;2-u

9.   Oregano: MedlinePlus Supplements. Medlineplus.gov. https://medlineplus.gov/druginfo/natural/644.html. Published 2018. Accessed August 14, 2018.

10.   3. Si H, Hu J, Liu Z, Zeng Z. Antibacterial effect of oregano essential oil alone and in combination with antibiotics against extended-spectrum β-lactamase-producing Escherichia coli: Table 1. *FEMS Immunology & Medical Microbiology*. 2008;53(2):190-194. doi:10.1111/j.1574-695x.2008.00414.x

Inflammation Control

Inflammation is a normal process meant to heal the body. However, it can get out of control and lead to major problems. Imagine running a marathon. When you finish, your knees will probably hurt, there may be some 'puffiness,' definitely stiffness and some collagen loss . Your natural inflammatory response will stimulate your body to begin healing itself. Within a week or so, you'll be fully recovered and likely even a little bit stronger than before. But imagine running that marathon *every day*. Your knees would *constantly* be experiencing inflammation and never be able to fully heal. In time, your tissues would break down and your knees would become far more painful, puffy and stiff. Pretty soon, no working knees! This is similar to what can happen inside your body! In fact, it is becoming more and more clear that *chronic inflammation* leads to disease.[1] Here are the 3 best supplements to reduce inflammation:

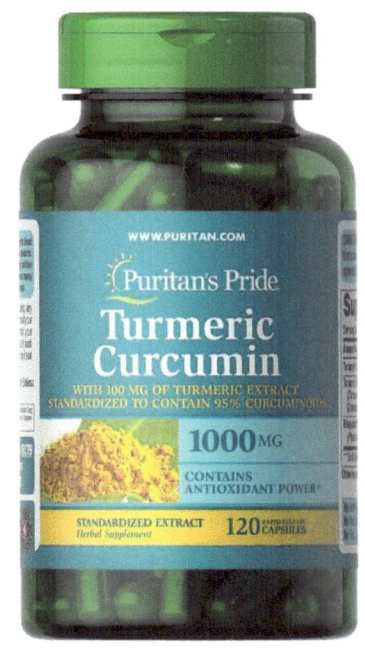

One of the Strongest Anti-Inflammatory Herbs

Many people are already familiar with turmeric because it is a popular spice, but it also has incredible health benefits. It is one of the best anti-inflammatory products out there. Plus it has powerful antioxidant properties.[2,3] In fact, it is so powerful that it combats all sorts of diseases of the heart and brain, fights diabetes, obesity, immune disorders, helps removes toxins and even fights cancer.[4,5,6,7,8,9,10,11] Keep in mind however, that turmeric *alone* is not very effective. It absorbs very poorly, but pipperine, from black pepper, can improve its absorption by as much as *2000%*.2 You can learn more *here* where I have written an entire article on turmeric.

Fish Oil and Inflammation

Fish oil has many benefits as well and is another of the most powerful natural anti-inflammatory supplements out there. Thus, it is *also* helpful in treating health problems such as heart disease, inflammatory bowel disease, arthritis and even cancer.[12] The benefits come from the omega 3's found in fish oil. These consist of DHA and EPA. Their amazing health protection was discovered years ago when we still thought *all* fat was bad. But researchers studying traditional Eskimos were baffled. These people eat a lot of seal and whale blubber, yet they almost never get heart disease or diabetes.[13]

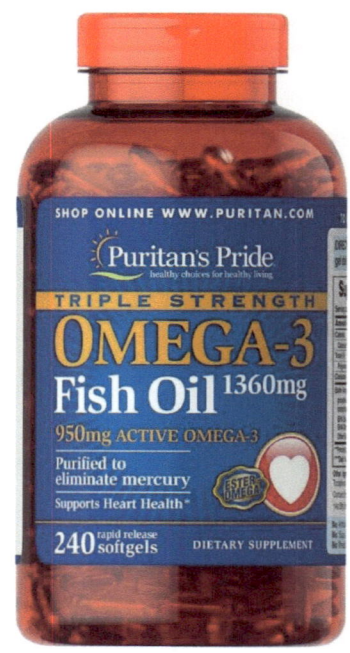

A Dose of Better Health with ALA

Alpha lipoic acid is another fat, similar to DHA and EPA that effectively reduce inflammation naturally. Insulin resistance, cancer, liver disease and heart disease are just a few of the health problems that ALA prevents.[14,15,16,17,18,19,20,21] Plus, it helps control blood sugar and diabetes.[23,24]

These alone are great reasons to take ALA, but there is more. It also protects cells from free radical damage as a powerful antioxidant.[22] But, it is not just a *regular* antioxidant. It is both fat and water soluble and can thus neutralize free radicals *anywhere* in your body. Most antioxidants, no matter how powerful, are *either* fat or water soluble, but not both.

Normally, free radicals can cause damage, referred to as oxidative stress. Oxidative stress causes significant inflammation. This leads to disease but antioxidants, especially ALA, eliminate these toxins before they can cause damage.

References

1.   Libby P. Inflammatory mechanisms: the molecular basis of inflammation and disease. Nutr Rev. 2007;65(12 Pt 2):S140-6.

2.   Hewlings SJ, Kalman DS. Curcumin: A Review of Its' Effects on Human Health. Foods. 2017;6(10)

3.   Abrahams S, Haylett WL, Johnson G, Carr JA, Bardien S. Antioxidant effects of curcumin in models of neurodegeneration, aging, oxidative and nitrosative stress: A review. Neuroscience. 2019;406:1-21.

4.   Sarraf P, Parohan M, Javanbakht MH, Ranji-burachaloo S, Djalali M. Short-term curcumin supplementation enhances serum brain-derived neurotrophic factor in adult men and women: a systematic review and dose-response meta-analysis of randomized controlled trials. Nutr Res. 2019;69:1-8.

5.   Haase J, Brown E. Integrating the monoamine, neurotrophin and cytokine hypotheses of depression–a central role for the serotonin transporter?. Pharmacol Ther. 2015;147:1-11.

6.   Qin XY, Cao C, Cawley NX, et al. Decreased peripheral brain-derived neurotrophic factor levels in Alzheimer's disease: a meta-analysis study (N=7277). Mol Psychiatry. 2017;22(2):312-320.

7.   Sanmukhani J, Satodia V, Trivedi J, et al. Efficacy and safety of curcumin in major depressive disorder: a randomized controlled trial. Phytother Res. 2014;28(4):579-85.

8.   Jiang S, Han J, Li T, et al. Curcumin as a potential protective compound against cardiac diseases. Pharmacol Res. 2017;119:373-383.

9.   Karimian MS, Pirro M, Johnston TP, Majeed M, Sahebkar A. Curcumin and Endothelial Function: Evidence and Mechanisms of Protective Effects. Curr Pharm Des. 2017;23(17):2462-2473.

10.   Kunnumakkara AB, Bordoloi D, Padmavathi G, et al. Curcumin, the golden nutraceutical: multitargeting for multiple chronic diseases. Br J Pharmacol. 2017;174(11):1325-1348.

11.   Shanmugam MK, Rane G, Kanchi MM, et al. The multifaceted role of curcumin in cancer prevention and treatment. Molecules. 2015;20(2):2728-69.

12.   Wall R, Ross R, Fitzgerald G, Stanton C. Fatty acids from fish: the anti-inflammatory potential of long-chain omega-3 fatty acids. *Nutr Rev*. 2010;68(5):280-289. doi:10.1111/j.1753-4887.2010.00287.x

13.   Nutrition classics. The Lancet, Vol. I for 1971: Plasma lipid and lipoprotein pattern in Greenlandic West-Coast Eskimos. By H.O. Bang, J. Dyerberg, Aase Brøndum Nielsen. Nutr Rev. 1986;44(4):143-6.

14.   Castro MC, Massa ML, Arbeláez LG, Schinella G, Gagliardino JJ, Francini F. Fructose-induced inflammation, insulin resistance and oxidative stress: A liver pathological triad effectively disrupted by lipoic acid. Life Sci. 2015;137:1-6.

15.   Moon HS. Chemopreventive Effects of Alpha Lipoic Acid on Obesity-Related Cancers. Ann Nutr Metab. 2016;68(2):137-44.

16.   Liu Z, Guo J, Sun H, Huang Y, Zhao R, Yang X. α-Lipoic acid attenuates LPS-induced liver injury by improving mitochondrial function in association with GR mitochondrial DNA occupancy. Biochimie. 2015;116:52-60.

17.   Sola S, Mir MQ, Cheema FA, et al. Irbesartan and lipoic acid improve endothelial function and reduce markers of inflammation in the metabolic syndrome: results of the Irbesartan and Lipoic Acid in Endothelial Dysfunction (ISLAND) study. Circulation. 2005;111(3):343-8.

18.   Khalili M, Azimi A, Izadi V, et al. Does lipoic acid consumption affect the cytokine profile in multiple sclerosis patients: a double-blind, placebo-controlled, randomized clinical trial. Neuroimmunomodulation. 2014;21(6):291-6.

19.   Han T, Bai J, Liu W, Hu Y. A systematic review and meta-analysis of α-lipoic acid in the treatment of diabetic peripheral neuropathy. Eur J Endocrinol. 2012;167(4):465-71.

20.   Hwang S, Byun JW, Yoon JS, Lee EJ. Inhibitory Effects of α-Lipoic Acid on Oxidative Stress-Induced Adipogenesis in Orbital Fibroblasts From Patients With Graves Ophthalmopathy. Medicine (Baltimore). 2016;95(2):e2497.

21.   Skibska B, Goraca A. The protective effect of lipoic acid on selected cardiovascular diseases caused by age-related oxidative stress. Oxid Med Cell Longev. 2015;2015:313021.

22.   Moura FA, De andrade KQ, Dos santos JC, Goulart MO. Lipoic Acid: its antioxidant and anti-inflammatory role and clinical applications. Curr Top Med Chem. 2015;15(5):458-83.

23.   Bashan N, Kovsan J, Kachko L, Ovadia H, Rudich A. Positive and negative regulation of insulin signaling by reactive oxygen and nitrogen species. Phys Rev. 2009;89(1):27-71.

24.   Morakinyo A, Awobajo FO, Adegoke OA. Effects of alpha lipoic acid on blood lipids, renal indices, antioxidant enzymes, insulin and glucose level in sereptozotocin-diabetic rats. Biol Med. Jan-Mar 2013(5.1):26.

Joint Relief

Throughout your body are many joints and that's a good thing since they allow you to move. Yet, they are easy to take for granted, of course until we get old and they start to hurt. Some folks assume this is a natural part of aging, but it doesn't have to be. Exercise helps of course and even avid runners have no more incidences of arthritis than non-runners, but they do have lower rates of muscular or skeletal disabilities.[1] But whether you exercise or not, you need an effective joint formula to keep your joints healthy so it doesn't hurt to simply move around!

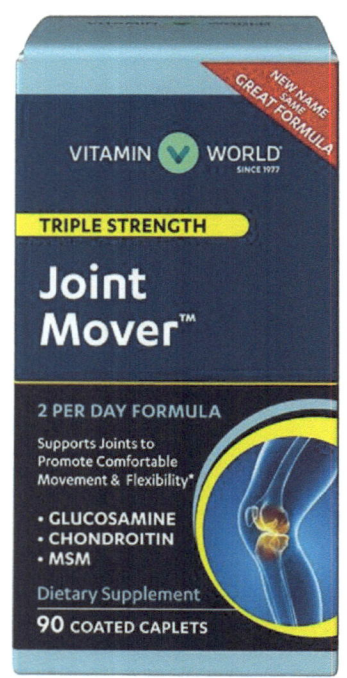

Glucosamine, Chondroitin, MSM

Surely you are familiar with glucosamine, chondroitin and maybe MSM and their use in joint strengthening products. Consequently, each can be found in Joint Mover™,a joint formula consisting of a complex of the three that helps build up new joint tissue and reduce pain. Because glucosamine and chondroitin literally make up what are called glycosaminoglycans, which are essentially what joints are made of, both are essential. Although your body makes some of these, consuming more can be beneficial as our body doesn't always do what we hope. In one study for example, participants were given a joint formula consisting of glucosamine. These individuals had less pain and healthier joints than those that did not.[2]

Likewise, similar results are found in studies with chondroitin.[3] MSM is another substance that is particularly beneficial for joints, although in larger doses it can relieve allergies too.[4] A naturally occurring source of sulfur, MSM has been shown to reduce pain and improve physical function in even short studies[5] and also provides even better benefits when combined with glucosamine.[6]

Bromelain

Bromelain comes from pineapple and is composed of various components that prevent edema, reduce the formation of blood clots, dissolve blood clots and reduce inflammation. It is also extremely safe with virtually no side effects and is even used as a complementary treatment for some cancers.[7] Because of its strong anti-inflammatory properties, bromelain is also an essential part of any joint formula. In fact, studies have shown that it can be an effective treatment in osteoarthritis[8] and proven to bestow positive benefits to bones and joints.[9]

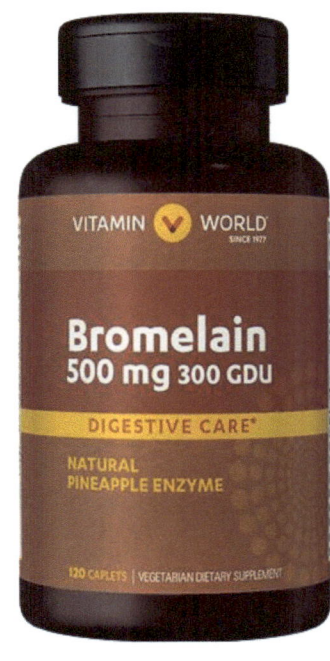

Fish Oil

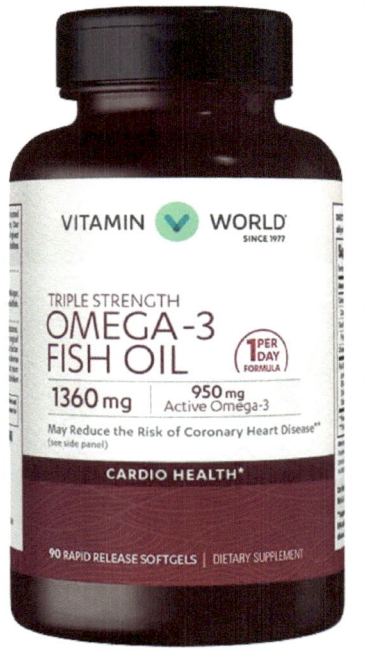

As you may have already noticed, fish oil helps with a lot of things because of its natural anti-inflammatory properties. Cardiovascular disease, inflammatory bowel disease, cancer and arthritis are all affected positively by the fats in fish oil because of this.[10] Inflammation is a natural immune response meant to protect the body, such as when your finger becomes red and swollen after you hit it with a hammer on accident.

The real problem occurs when this response becomes chronic, or ongoing. Your finger eventually gets better and is back to normal but imagine if it never did. You would end up with serious finger problems eventually, namely the breakdown of internal tissue, which is the ultimate result of chronic inflammation.[11] Consequently, your joints are no different and that is why fish oil should be part of any good joint formula. When they become inflamed, which they will, it will lead to arthritis and eventually all the pain and immobility associated with it. However, taking fish oil can significantly reduce your risk and keep your joints feeling much better along the way.[12]

References

1.   Publishing H. Exercise and your joints – Harvard Health. Harvard Health.

https://www.health.harvard.edu/newsletter_article/exercise-and-your-joints. Published 2018. Accessed August 15,

2018.

2.   Reginster J, Deroisy R, Rovati L et al. Long-term effects of glucosamine sulphate on osteoarthritis

progression: a randomised, placebo-controlled clinical trial. *The Lancet*. 2001;357(9252):251-256.

doi:10.1016/s0140-6736(00)03610-2

3.   McAlindon T, LaValley M, Gulin J, Felson D. Glucosamine and Chondroitin for Treatment of

Osteoarthritis. *JAMA*. 2000;283(11):1469. doi:10.1001/jama.283.11.1469

4.   Barrager E, Veltmann J, Schauss A, Schiller R. A Multicentered, Open-Label Trial on the Safety and

Efficacy of Methylsulfonylmethane in the Treatment of Seasonal Allergic Rhinitis. *The Journal of Alternative and

Complementary Medicine*. 2002;8(2):167-173. doi:10.1089/107555302317371451

5.   Kim L, Axelrod L, Howard P, Buratovich N, Waters R. Efficacy of methylsulfonylmethane (MSM) in

osteoarthritis pain of the knee: a pilot clinical trial. *Osteoarthr Cartil*. 2006;14(3):286-294.

doi:10.1016/j.joca.2005.10.003

6.   Usha P, Naidu M. Randomised, Double-Blind, Parallel, Placebo-Controlled Study of Oral Glucosamine,

Methylsulfonylmethane and their Combination in Osteoarthritis. *Clin Drug Investig*. 2004;24(6):353-363.

doi:10.2165/00044011-200424060-00005

7.   Maurer H. Bromelain: biochemistry, pharmacology and medical use. *Cellular and Molecular Life Sciences*.

2001;58(9):1234-1245. doi:10.1007/pl00000936

8.   Brien S, Lewith G, Walker A, Hicks S, Middleton D. Bromelain as a Treatment for Osteoarthritis: a

Review of Clinical Studies. *Evidence-Based Complementary and Alternative Medicine*. 2004;1(3):251-257.

doi:10.1093/ecam/neh035

9.   Cicero A, Colletti A. Nutraceuticals Active on Bones and Joints. *Handbook of Nutraceuticals for Clinical

Use*. 2018:181-193. doi:10.1007/978-3-319-73642-6_14

10.   Wall R, Ross R, Fitzgerald G, Stanton C. Fatty acids from fish: the anti-inflammatory potential of long-chain omega-3 fatty acids. *Nutr Rev*. 2010;68(5):280-289. doi:10.1111/j.1753-4887.2010.00287.x

11.   Bhatt D. What is inflammation? – Harvard Health. Harvard Health. https://www.health.harvard.edu/heart-disease-overview/ask-the-doctor-what-is-inflammation. Published 2017. Accessed August 25, 2018.

12.   Felson D, Bischoff-Ferrari H. Dietary fatty acids for the treatment of OA, including fish oil. *Ann Rheum Dis*. 2015;75(1):1-2. doi:10.1136/annrheumdis-2015-208329

Kid's Health

The nutritional needs of children are really not that much different than that of their parents. Aren't they just mini adults after all? A kid's health still requires the same basic nutrients including fats, proteins, carbohydrates, vitamins and minerals, but the proportion of each they need will vary some depending on their age and gender. They are growing and so their needs not only include what their body requires to continue functioning normally, but also some beyond that for growth.[1]

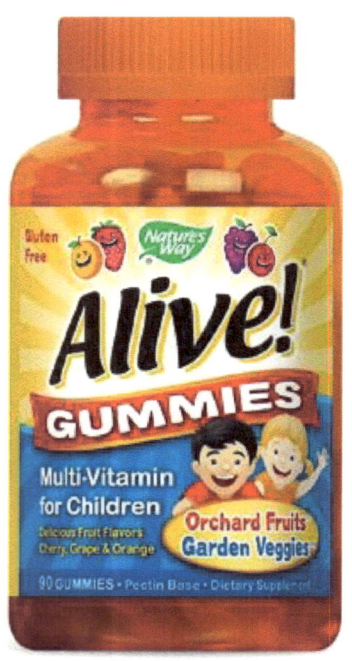

Chewable Multivitamin

Everyone should take a multivitamin to ensure they are getting all the vitamins and minerals they need, especially kids. They are growing *and* performing the processes of life at a greater rate than adults and failure to receive sufficient nutrition, like not getting enough iodine, can result in stunted growth.[2] It is ironic that often we pay little attention to kid's health while we take our vitamins. And yet we aren't even growing! Children are, and thus need additional nutrition that much more to fulfill the cellular needs of life as well as growth.

Chewable C

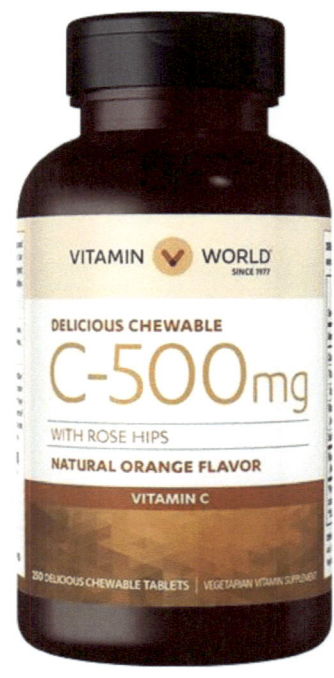

If you read the immune system entry you already know that there are a great many benefits to taking vitamin C. These of course apply to children as well. So, don't we want to boost their immune system and reduce disease risk in them too? Of course we do! These are wonderful benefits to vitamin C, but we especially cannot forget that it is also essential in the production of collagen.[3,4] Children (of course) are producing new tissues all the time, after all, that's what growing is, and that means lots of collagen, which means lots of vitamin C.

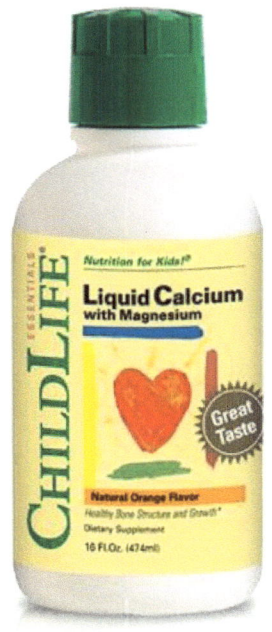

Liquid Calcium/Magnesium

If you've ever been a parent then you know that kids grow like weeds, which requires bones that grow like weeds. Obviously to grow taller one must increase bone length, which requires collagen, proteins, and of course calcium. I explained in the bone health section, that when the body doesn't have enough calcium in the bloodstream then it robs it from bone.[5,6] This is a really bad thing for a kid's health since their bones can potentially end up less than as sturdy as they ought to be. But just like adults, magnesium and vitamin D are also essential to ensure that calcium is absorbed properly so as to be useful.[7]

References

1.   Mayo Clinic Staff. What nutrients does your child need now?. Mayo Clinic. https://www.mayoclinic.org/healthy-lifestyle/childrens-health/in-depth/nutrition-for-kids/art-20049335. Published 2018. Accessed August 27, 2018.

2.   Engle P, Black M, Behrman J et al. Strategies to avoid the loss of developmental potential in more than 200 million children in the developing world. *The Lancet*. 2007;369(9557):229-242.

3.   Office of Dietary Supplements – Vitamin C. Ods.od.nih.gov. https://ods.od.nih.gov/factsheets/VitaminC-HealthProfessional/. Published 2018. Accessed July 27, 2018.

4.   Wilson J. Mechanism of action of vitamin C in sepsis: Ascorbate modulates redox signaling in endothelium. BioFactors. 2009;35(1):5-13. doi:10.1002/biof.7 doi:10.1016/s0140-6736(07)60112-3

5.   Wisse B, David Z. What causes bone loss? : MedlinePlus Medical Encyclopedia. *Medlineplusgov*. 2016. Available at: https://medlineplus.gov/ency/patientinstructions/000506.htm. Accessed June 21, 2018.

6.   Drugs & Medications. *Webmdcom*. 2018. Available at: https://www.webmd.com/drugs/2/drug-64799/coral-calcium-oral/details. Accessed June 21, 2018.

7.   Nutrition's dynamic duos – Harvard Health. Harvard Health. 2009. Available at: https://www.health.harvard.edu/newsletter_article/Nutritions-dynamic-duos. Accessed June 21, 2018.

Liver Safety

More people than you might think experience liver damage. Just consider that its job is essentially to filter out all the "crap" in your blood. And while it's a rather large organ, you've only got one. Disease is typically progressive, beginning with steatosis. In layman's terms, 'some damage,' but not too serious. Enough damage becomes hepatitis and parts of it become fibrous and no longer function. Next is cirrhosis and then hepatocellular carcinoma (that's cancer).[1]

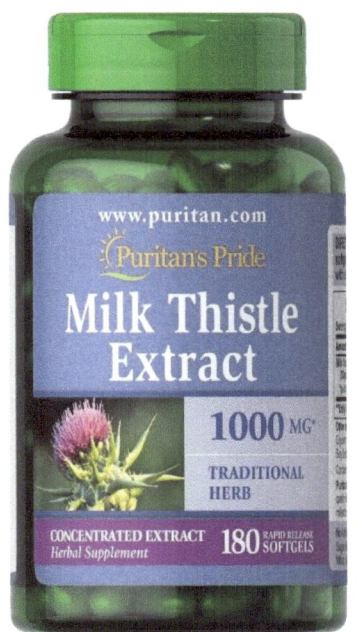

Milk Thistle

Milk thistle is an herb that has been in use for thousands of years. It is still in use as a common way to help detoxify the liver. The effective ingredient is called *Silybum marianum* but is often just called silymarin. Studies have shown that milk thistle extracts fight cancer and diabetes and improve heart health. In addition, it shows promise in the fight against liver disease, cancer, hepatitis, HIV, and high cholesterol. It is also well tolerated and safe.[2]

Lycopene

Tomatoes are a very abundant source of lycopene, particularly in the Western diet. It is a powerful antioxidant that neutralizes free radicals that might otherwise cause damage. Antioxidants in general have been proposed for treatment of liver disorders and some seem to help. But lycopene has proven to be the most effective while some others have shown mixed results.[3]

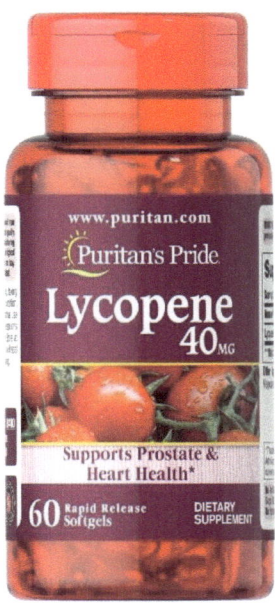

Zinc for Strong Functioning

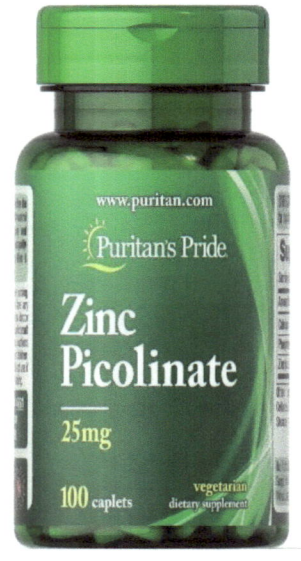

Another effective supplement is zinc. It is an essential mineral necessary for cells to divide and form new DNA. You can imagine how important this process is in the liver where there is constant turnover of cells. In fact, studies have found a strong link between low zinc levels of zinc and liver diseases. In short, if you want to retain a healthy liver or already have problems, zinc is essential.[4] Also know that not all forms of zinc are equal. Some absorb better than others and zinc picolinate is one of the best.

References

1.   Vitaglione P, Morisco F, Caporaso N, Fogliano V. Dietary antioxidant compounds and liver health. Critical Reviews in Food Science and Nutrition. 2005;44(7-8):575-586.

2.   Tamayo C, Diamond S. Review of clinical trials evaluating safety and efficacy of milk thistle(silybum marianum[l.] gaertn.). Integr Cancer Ther. 2007;6(2):146-157.

3.   Vitaglione P, Morisco F, Caporaso N, Fogliano V. Dietary antioxidant compounds and liver health. Critical Reviews in Food Science and Nutrition. 2005;44(7-8):575-586.

4.   Mohammad MK, Zhou Z, Cave M, Barve A, McClain CJ. Zinc and liver disease. Nutr Clin Pract. 2012;27(1):8-20.

Male Fitness

It is easy to get caught up in the political correctness of our world and not realize that male health needs are as significant as their female counterparts. Politics aside, the fact of the matter is that men are different than women. On average, men have higher base metabolic rates, differing skeletal structures, different size organs, slower hearts and significantly more powerful muscles.[1] Now all this simply means that a man has different nutritional needs.

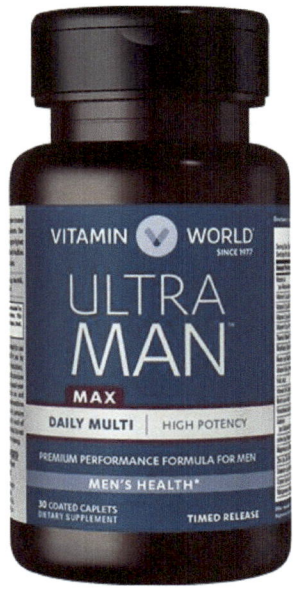

Multivitamin

A multivitamin provides a wellness insurance policy for male health. As a man, it helps ensure that you have all the essential vitamins and minerals that your body needs. While you may often hear that a well-rounded diet eliminates the need for a multivitamin, which it does in principle, the fact of the matter is that most people just don't get what they need every day.[2] This formula is not only made to meet your specific male health needs, but it is also 'time-release,' meaning it delivers a small, steady stream of nutrients over a longer period of time.

Prostate Healthy

The prostate glands are particularly important for men because so much can go wrong with them. At the time of this writing, it is expected that this year, nearly 10% of all new cancer cases will be of the prostate and 30,000 people will die of it.3 Fortunately, much can be done! The ingredients in the Advanced Prostate Formula improve the health of the prostate and reduce your risk of cancer. For example, lycopene and selenium are just two of the ingredients that have shown to reduce your risk.4,5 Others such as saw palmetto and pumpkin seed are also commonly associated with prostate health.

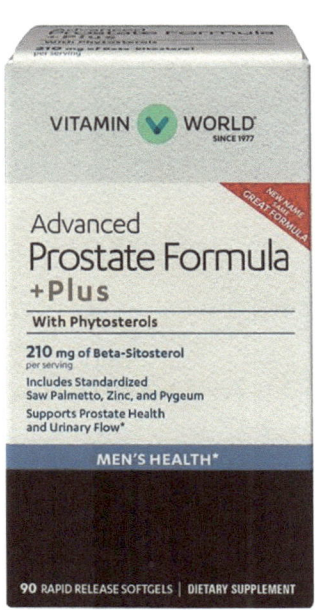

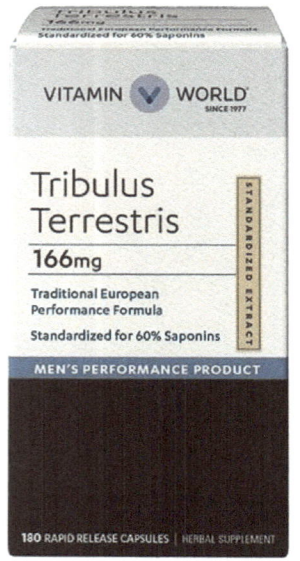

Testosterone

Testosterone is the hormone that makes a man a man. It is also the reason that men tend to be more muscular, aggressive and sex-driven than women.[6] But testosterone levels are not only necessary to support male health. They are all associated with overall wellness. For example, low testosterone increases your risk of type-2 diabetes as well as prostate cancer.[7,8] Furthermore, sufficient testosterone levels decline with age, so keeping them up becomes more and more important over time, especially when you consider that aging negatively affects testosterone levels as much as poor health and lifestyle.[9] Tribulus terrestris is an herb that is known to effectively increase testosterone in men and thus improve male health.[10]

References

1.   Dobson, J. (2018). The Physical Differences Between Women and Me. Retrieved from https://www.dobsonlibrary.com/resource/article/9149f0c1-006e-4e69-8443-f4901c11843e

2.   Angelo G, Drake V, Frei B. Efficacy of Multivitamin/mineral Supplementation to Reduce Chronic Disease Risk: A Critical Review of the Evidence from Observational Studies and Randomized Controlled Trials. Crit Rev Food Sci Nutr. 2014;55(14):1968-1991. doi:10.1080/10408398.2014.912199

3.   Prostate Cancer – Cancer Stat Facts. Seer.cancer.gov. https://seer.cancer.gov/statfacts/html/prost.html. Published 2018. Accessed September 11, 2018.

4.   Wertz K, Siler U, Goralczyk R. Lycopene: modes of action to promote prostate health. Arch Biochem Biophys. 2004;430(1):127-134. doi:10.1016/j.abb.2004.04.023

5.   Clark L, Dalkin B, Krongrad A et al. Decreased incidence of prostate cancer with selenium supplementation: results of a double-blind cancer prevention trial. BJU Int. 1998;81(5):730-734. doi:10.1046/j.1464-410x.1998.00630.x

6.   Harrison W. Understanding How Testosterone Affects Men. National Institutes of Health (NIH). https://www.nih.gov/news-events/nih-research-matters/understanding-how-testosterone-affects-men. Published 2013. Accessed September 12, 2018.

7.   Selvin, E., Feinleib, M., Zhang, L., Rohrmann, S., Rifai, N., & Nelson, W. et al. (2007). Androgens and Diabetes in Men: Results from the Third National Health and Nutrition Examination Survey (NHANES III). Diabetes Care, 30(2), 234-238. doi: 10.2337/dc06-1579

8.   Schatzl G, Madersbacher S, Thurridl T et al. High-grade prostate cancer is associated with low serum testosterone levels. Prostate. 2001;47(1):52-58. doi:10.1002/pros.1046

9.   Travison T, Araujo A, Kupelian V, O'Donnell A, McKinlay J. The Relative Contributions of Aging, Health, and Lifestyle Factors to Serum Testosterone Decline in Men. The Journal of Clinical Endocrinology & Metabolism. 2007;92(2):549-555. doi:10.1210/jc.2006-1859

10.   Chhatre S, Nesari T, Kanchan D, Somani G, Sathaye S. Phytopharmacological overview of Tribulus terrestris. Pharmacogn Rev. 2014;8(15):45. doi:10.4103/0973-7847.125530

Muscle Training

When it comes to supplements for building larger muscles, nothing can replace adequate training and diet. Sorry to disappoint, but there is no magic bullet. In other words, you have to train and eat properly too. Then, and only then is it even worth taking supplements because at that point they do provide positive results. For example, a recent study found that when people who had started a resistance training program who did not seem to benefit from protein supplementation, and then moved up their volume, frequency and duration, saw significant benefit.[1] So by all means, supplements can help you build bigger muscles. But they will not and cannot replace lazy training or inadequate protein or calories.

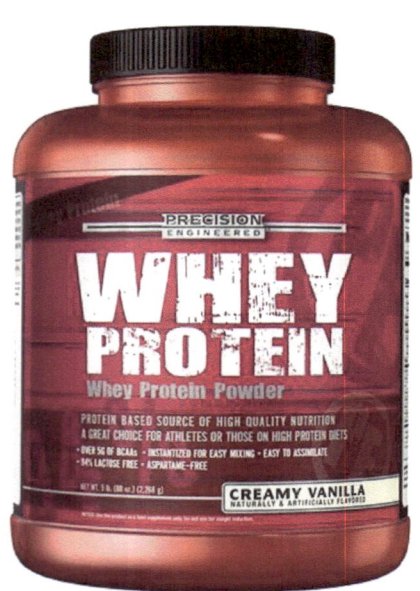

Whey Protein

Much of what will determine your muscle building will happen shortly after your workout as a result of what type of protein you consume. However, whey protein is special in its ability to absorb quickly and promote muscle growth more so than other forms. Consequently, this means that it can get into your bloodstream and to your muscles as quickly as possible to start building more tissue. Although your body can make some amino acids, three of the ones that it can't happen to be very important in the construction of muscle tissue and happen to be abundant in whey. These are known as the branch chain amino acids; leucine, isoleucine and valine.[2] Of course drinking a whey protein shake is a great way to get extra protein anytime, it is especially important to consume at least 50 grams right after each workout.

Creatine

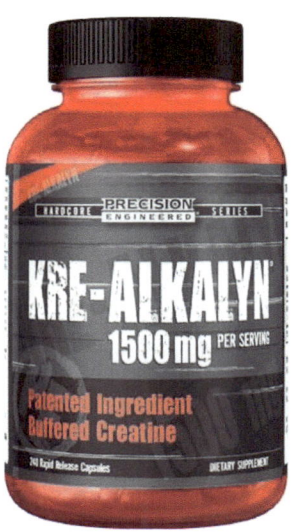

Creatine sometimes strikes fear into people, especially parents of teenage boys and is often mistakenly associated with illegal performance enhancing drugs. Although we might speculate about where these ideas come from, the truth is that creatine has failed to produce significant side effect aside from supporting the growth of muscles[3] Creatine is found almost exclusively in muscle tissue and in effect, 'recycles' energy that is turned over rapidly during lifting, ultimately providing the user with a greater muscular capacity.[4] Lifting weights, when done properly, requires an explosion of energy and creatine effectively increases that amount of time that explosion can last and reduces recovery time between sets.

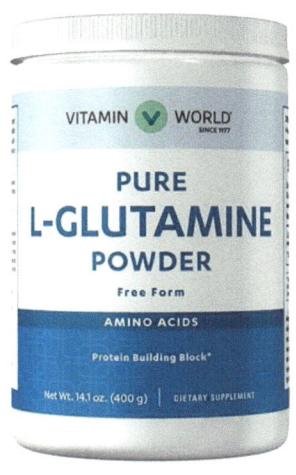

Glutamine

There are a total of 20 amino acids that make up human protein, but only about half of them are necessary in your diet and your body can make the rest.[5] However, of all of them, glutamine is the most abundant amino acid in the entire body as well as in muscle tissue.[6] Because of this, glutamine has been shown to significantly enhance muscle growth following strength training, lower rates of soreness and also decrease recovery times.[7]

References

1.   Pasiakos S, McLellan T, Lieberman H. The Effects of Protein Supplements on Muscle Mass, Strength, and Aerobic and Anaerobic Power in Healthy Adults: A Systematic Review. *Sports Medicine*. 2014;45(1):111-131. doi:10.1007/s40279-014-0242-2

2.   Devries M, Phillips S. Supplemental Protein in Support of Muscle Mass and Health: Advantage Whey. *J Food Sci*. 2015;80(S1):A8-A15. doi:10.1111/1750-3841.12802

3.   Jäger R, Purpura M, Shao A, Inoue T, Kreider R. Analysis of the efficacy, safety, and regulatory status of novel forms of creatine. *Amino Acids*. 2011;40(5):1369-1383. doi:10.1007/s00726-011-0874-6

4.   Volek J, Kraemer W. Creatine Supplementation. *J Strength Cond Res*. 1996;10(3):200-210. doi:10.1519/00124278-199608000-00014

5.   Marieb E, Keller S. *Essentials Of Human Anatomy & Physiology*. 10th ed. San Francisco: Pearson Education Inc.; :490.

6.   de Vasconcelos M, Tirapegui J. Nutritional Importance of Glutamine. *PubMed*. 1998;35(3):207-215. PMID:10029867

7.   Legault Z, Bagnall N, Kimmerly D. The Influence of Oral L-Glutamine Supplementation on Muscle Strength Recovery and Soreness Following Unilateral Knee Extension Eccentric Exercise. *Int J Sport Nutr Exerc Metab*. 2015;25(5):417-426. doi:10.1123/ijsnem.2014-0209

Sleep Soundly

Since we live in a fast-paced world, it often feels like we just can't afford 8 hours of sleep a night. But the truth is that getting the proper amount of rest EVERY night is essential to your health.[1] You can exercise and eat right, but if you are tired all the time, you are still at risk. Consequently, chronic fatigue can wreak havoc on your metabolism. It also causes damage to DNA, accelerate aging and increase inflammation (a marker for increased cancer risk).[2,3,4]

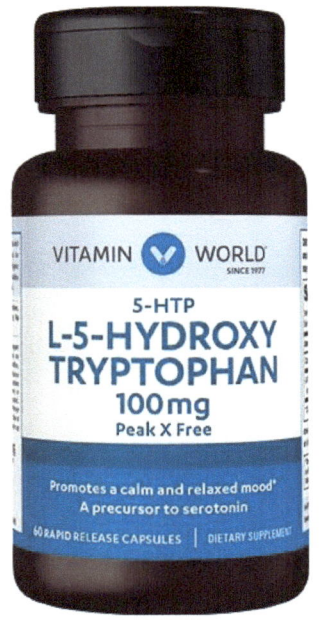

5-HTP (Hydroxy-tryptophan)

5-HTP is short for *5-hydroxytryptophan* and is a precursor to the neurotransmitter serotonin. Thus, you must have it to make seratonin.[5] However, your body can and does form 5-HTP using the amino acid tryptophan. It is abundant in animal protein, particularly turkey, but tryptophan alone will not make you feel tired, although a full stomach can. Of course, it also regulates brain activities that include getting to and staying asleep.[6] So unless your body is does a perfect job at making 5-HTP, you could benefit from supplementing with it. Consequently, few bodies do a perfect job at this and they become less efficient with age.

Melatonin

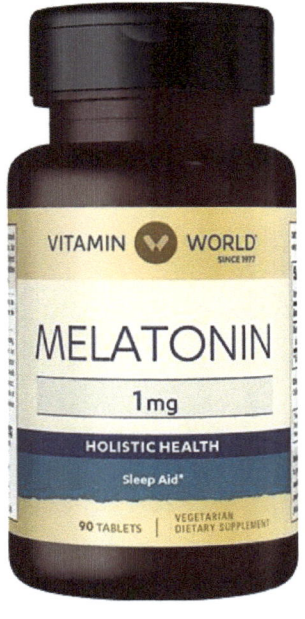

Melatonin is a hormone that is produced in the brain where its role is to regulate your rest cycles. As you might expect, it increases in the dark and decreases during the daytime, which is why some folks have such a hard time getting enough rest when they work nights. Nonetheless, several studies have shown that melatonin is effective in treating many of these disorders including insomnia and jet lag and may even help with Alzheimers.[7] In any case natural melatonin production decreases with age. So even if you are in good overall health, you may be having trouble sleeping simply because your body does not produce as much melatonin as it used to.[8] In short, children, especially teenagers, sleep like bears during hibernation! Yet as adults as many as 50% of us struggle to fall asleep, stay asleep and feel fully rested afterwards.[9]

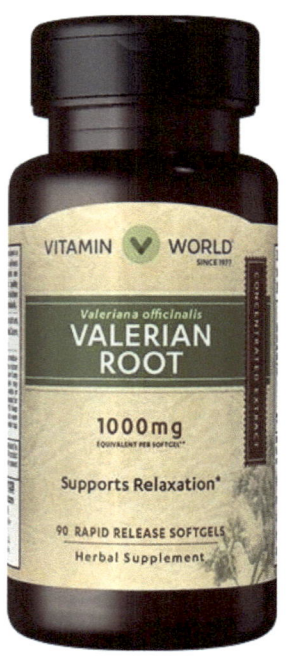

Valerian

Valerian root is an herb, typically found in dietary supplements. It is also a common ingredient in over the counter medications. While it is not clear why valerian works, it has been shown to have sedative effects. There is also very little risk associated with consumption of valerian. Unlike many drugs out there, valerian does not cause side effects that are arguably worse than being tired![10] Many studies have illustrated just how effective valerian can be at inducing sleep as well as improving its quality.[11] Moreover, some of the ladies out there will find a bonus to taking valerian. Consequently, it has been shown to reduce emotional, physical and behavioral symptoms associated with premenstrual syndrome.[12]

References

1.   Mukherjee S, Patel S, Kales S et al. An Official American Thoracic Society Statement: The Importance of Healthy Sleep. Recommendations and Future Priorities. *Am J Respir Crit Care Med*. 2015;191(12):1450-1458. doi:10.1164/rccm.201504-0767st

2.   Kushida C. *Sleep Deprivation*. New York: Marcel Dekker; 2005.

3.   Carroll J, Cole S, Seeman T et al. Partial sleep deprivation activates the DNA damage response (DDR) and the senescence-associated secretory phenotype (SASP) in aged adult humans. *Brain Behav Immun*. 2016;51:223-229. doi:10.1016/j.bbi.2015.08.024

4.   Irwin M, Olmstead R, Carroll J. Sleep Disturbance, Sleep Duration, and Inflammation: A Systematic Review and Meta-Analysis of Cohort Studies and Experimental Sleep Deprivation. *Biol Psychiatry*. 2016;80(1):40-52. doi:10.1016/j.biopsych.2015.05.014

5.   Zhang H, Zhao H, Yang X, Xue Q, Cotten J, Feng H. 5-Hydroxytryptophan, a precursor for serotonin synthesis, reduces seizure-induced respiratory arrest. *Epilepsia*. 2016;57(8):1228-1235. doi:10.1111/epi.13430

6.   Cespuglio R. Serotonin: its place today in sleep preparation, triggering or maintenance. *Sleep Med*. 2018;49:31-39.

7.   Staff. Melatonin. Mayo Clinic. https://www.mayoclinic.org/drugs-supplements-melatonin/art-20363071. Published 2018. Accessed September 25, 2018

8.   Zeitzer J, Duffy J, Lockley S, Dijk D, Czeisler C. Plasma Melatonin Rhythms In Young and Older Humans During Sleep, Sleep Deprivation, and Wake. *Sleep*. 2007;30(11):1437-1443.

9.   Crowley K. Sleep and Sleep Disorders in Older Adults. *Neuropsychol Rev*. 2011;21(1):41-53. doi:10.1007/s11065-010-9154-6

10.   Staff. Office of Dietary Supplements – Valerian. Ods.od.nih.gov. https://ods.od.nih.gov/factsheets/Valerian-HealthProfessional/. Published 2013. Accessed September 29, 2018.

11.   Bent S, Padula A, Moore D, Patterson M, Mehling W. Valerian for Sleep: A Systematic Review and Meta-Analysis. *Am J Med*. 2006;119(12):1005-1012. doi:10.1016/j.amjmed.2006.02.026

12.   Behboodi Moghadam Z, Rezaei E, Shirood Gholami R, Kheirkhah M, Haghani H. The effect of Valerian root extract on the severity of pre menstrual syndrome symptoms. *J Tradit Complement Med*. 2016;6(3):309-315. doi:10.1016/j.jtcme.2015.09.001

Stress Less

Stress comes in many forms and a little is good, but a lot is not-so-much. As a result of various stressor, the body will suffer. Consequently, it doesn't even matter if the stress is real or perceived. For example, you might be overwhelmed just because you think you might lose your job even if it is quite secure. Moreover, too much stress can lead to all sorts of emotional, psychological and emotional problems. As it turns out, anxiety is experienced by the brain, but the manifestations occur in the body. For example, you might experience headaches, high blood pressure, dry mouth, grinding teeth and so on.[1] Thus, ensuring that your brain has the nutrients it requires to manage stress effectively is paramount to your sanity!

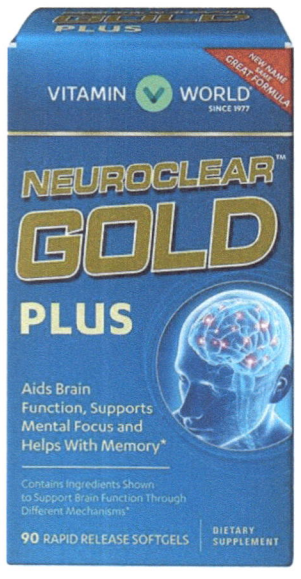

Phosphatidylserine

Every cell in your body is surrounded by a membrane composed of phospholipids (a special type of fat) and a little bit of protein, carbohydrates and cholesterol. In fact, his membrane is a lot like the front door of your home. Above all, its job is to keep good stuff in and bad stuff out. It just so happens that in your brain cells, one of these phospholipids, called phosphatidylserine (or PS), is the most common.[2] Thus, if you always have enough PS, you better ensure that your brain is able to manage stress effectively . In fact, PS supplementation has been shown to have a positive effect on stress as well as some of the problems associated with it such as poor memory and inability to focus.[3,4]

S-Adenosylmethionine (SAM-e)

SAM-e is found naturally in the body that helps maintain the membranes of cells and regulate hormones, which can be thrown out of whack in the presence of too much stress. Of course, hormones gone awry never results in effective stress management! Consequently, most people that experience depression display low levels

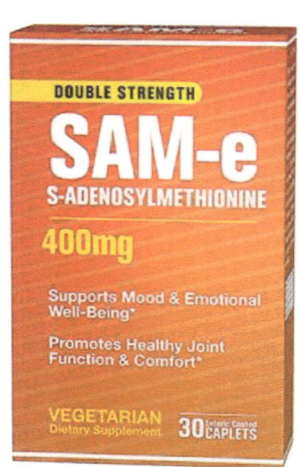

of serotonin, dopamine and norepinephrine. All of these neurotransmitters are associated with mental health and SAM-e not only slows their breakdown so they work longer, but also increase receptor sensitivity to them. In addition, research confirms that those who supplement with SAM-e have higher levels of all 3 of these brain chemicals among depressed and non-depressed patients alike.[5]

Gamma-Aminobutyric Acid

Gamma-aminobutyric acid, or GABA for short, plays a major role in the stress response of the brain.[6] Because it functions directly in the brain cells to mediate neurotransmitters (the chemicals the brain uses to communicate), it directly affects how you feel. GABA and glutamate, an amino acid, work together to create a balance between an excited and inhibitory response in brain cells. When a lack of GABA exists, normal signaling is interrupted and the brain cells don't respond quite right. Consequently, this can manifest itself in anxiety disorders and even

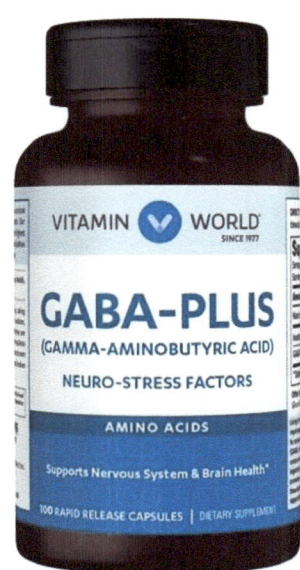

phobias.[7] Brain chemistry is essentially always the cause of depression, anxiety and other mental disorders. Thus, ensuring that the brain has the proper nutrients to function properly is paramount to ensuring that your body is able to manage stress effectively.

References

1.   Karriem-Norwood V. Stress Symptoms: Effects of Stress on the Body. WebMD. https://www.webmd.com/balance/stress-management/stress-symptoms-effects_of-stress-on-the-body#1. Published 2017. Accessed December 2, 2018.

2.   Alberts B. *Molecular Biology Of The Cell*. 6th ed. New York, NY [u.a.]: Garland Science; 2015.

3.   *Phosphatidylserine. Uofmhealthorg*. 2015. Available at: https://www.uofmhealth.org/health-library/hn-2896001. Accessed June 22, 2018.

4.   Hellhammer J, Vogt D, Franz N, Freitas U, Rutenberg D. A soy-based phosphatidylserine/ phosphatidic acid complex (PAS) normalizes the stress reactivity of hypothalamus-pituitary-adrenal-axis in chronically stressed

male subjects: a randomized, placebo-controlled study. *Lipids Health Dis*. 2014;13(1):121. doi:10.1186/1476-511x-13-121

5.   Olson S. Integrative Therapies for Depression – Serotonin Precursors – SAMe. Mentalhelp.net. https://www.mentalhelp.net/articles/integrative-therapies-for-depression-serotonin-precursors-same/. Published 2018. Accessed December 2, 2018.

6.   Herman J, Mueller N, Figueiredo H. Role of GABA and Glutamate Circuitry in Hypothalamo-Pituitary-Adrenocortical Stress Integration. *Ann N Y Acad Sci*. 2004;1018(1):35-45. doi:10.1196/annals.1296.004

7.   Milosevic I, McCabe R. *Phobias*. Santa Barbara, California: Greenwood, an imprint of ABC-CLIO, LLC; 2015.

Weight Loss

Many of us want to lose weight, but a lot of us fail at dieting for a number of reasons. There are two big ones when it comes to supplements. First, you may feel like a good diet pill is *cheating* somehow and forgo the benefits that some supplements can provide. Second, you may expect the supplement to do the work *for* you. You think (or blindly hope) that you don't have to watch what you eat or start exercising, supposing that the pill will, or should, magically melt the pounds away. Consequently, both are incorrect. Surely you should consider supplements to help you shed unwanted weight because they will enhance your efforts. However, understand that a good diet pill will only **help** you in your weight loss efforts. It will not make up for a poor diet or low activity level.[1] Even great supplements will not have much effect in the absence of calorie control and exercise.

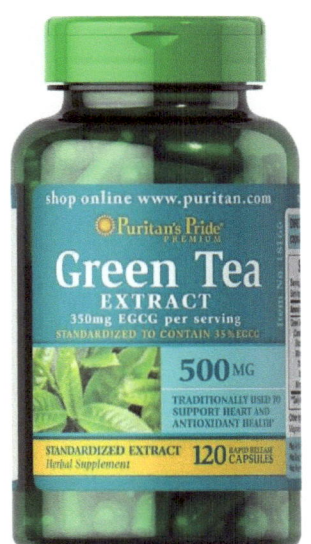

Thermogenics

This is one of the most effective healthy weight loss pills for boosting your metabolism. When your metabolism increases, you burn more calories than you did before. Of course, the most important calories you burn include fat stores. Caffeine and green tea are two effective ingredients that have been shown to encourage weight loss.[2] Ironically, green tea contains caffeine. This is a must-have in a supplemental arsenal for weight loss.

Conjugated Linoleic Acid (CLA)

Short for conjugated linoleic acid, CLA is a type of fatty acid that is occurs naturally in beef and dairy products. It has proven to an effective weight loss aid and also increases insulin sensitivity, decrease blood sugar, fights toxins and even may help with atherosclerosis. Scientists believe that the reason it makes for such a good diet pill is that it promotes apoptosis in fat cells. In other words, CLA encourages fat cells to kill themselves.[3] This is particularly significant because the number of fat

56

cells in your body is essentially fixed in childhood.[4] Therefore, staying thin becomes a little bit easier with fewer places for fat to hide.

Glucomannan

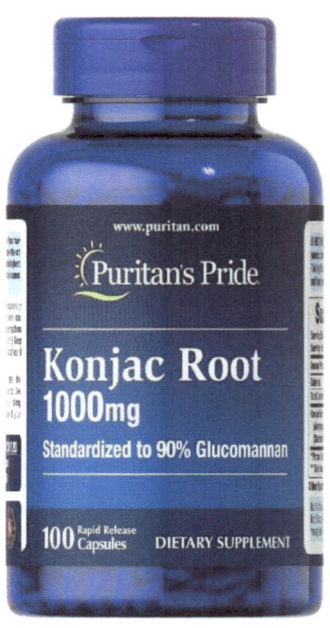

This formula contains konjac root, or elephant yam, a natural source of a special type of fiber called glucomannan. It is very unique in its ability to absorb enormous amounts of liquid, which is why it is such a good weight loss aid. First, glucomannan makes up about 40% of konjac, so it is naturally very low in calories. Second, it takes up a lot of space in your stomach, so you feel full with less food. Thirdly, it delays the emptying of the stomach which also contributes to feeling full longer. Fourth, it slows digestion and thus the amount of calories your body can absorb in a given time. Lastly, it is a food source for the friendly bacteria in your gut. A healthy bacterial landscape has also been associated with effective weight loss.[5]

References

1. Johns D, Hartmann-Boyce J, Jebb S, Aveyard P. *Diet or Exercise Interventions vs Combined Behavioral Weight Management Programs: A Systematic Review and Meta-Analysis of Direct Comparisons*. J Acad Nutr Diet. 2014;114(10):1557-1568. doi:10.1016/j.jand.2014.07.005

2. Westerterp-Plantenga M, Lejeune M, Kovacs E. *Body Weight Loss and Weight Maintenance in Relation to Habitual Caffeine* Intake and Green Tea Supplementation. Obes Res. 2005;13(7):1195-1204. doi:10.1038/oby.2005.142

3. Egras A, Hamilton W, Lenz T, Monaghan M. *An Evidence-Based Review of Fat Modifying Supplemental* Weight Loss *Products*. J Obes. 2011;2011:1-7. doi:10.1155/2011/297315

4. Hopkin M. *Fat cell numbers stay constant through adult life*. Nature. 2008. doi:10.1038/news.2008.800

5.   Arnarson A. *Glucomannan — Is It an Effective* Weight Loss *Supplement?*.

Healthline. https://www.healthline.com/nutrition/glucomannan. Published 2018. Accessed December 6, 2018.

Women's Wellness

Politics aside, the fact of the matter is that women are different than men and thus have unique nutritional needs. While women may have some physical 'disadvantages' compared to men, they dominate in other important ways, including a longer lifespan and ability to survive through adverse conditions.[1] Now all this simply means that a man has different nutritional needs.

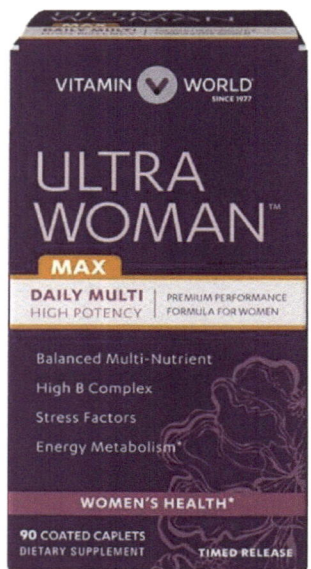

Multivitamin

A multivitamin provides a wellness insurance policy for female health. As a woman, it helps ensure that you have all the essential vitamins and minerals that your body needs. While you may often hear that a well-rounded diet eliminates the need for a multivitamin, which it does in principle, the fact of the matter is that most people just don't get what they need every day.[2] This formula is not only made to meet your specific female health needs, but it is also 'time-release,' meaning it delivers a small, steady stream of nutrients throughout the day.

Fish Oil

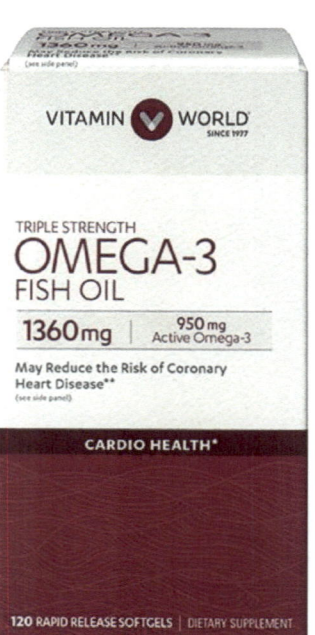

Fish oil is a great supplement for about a million reasons, but for women, it contributes to the health of skin, hair and nails. The DHA and EPA in fish oil are hard to find anywhere else and are essential for the body. They literally function as anti-aging components.[3]

Retinol Cream

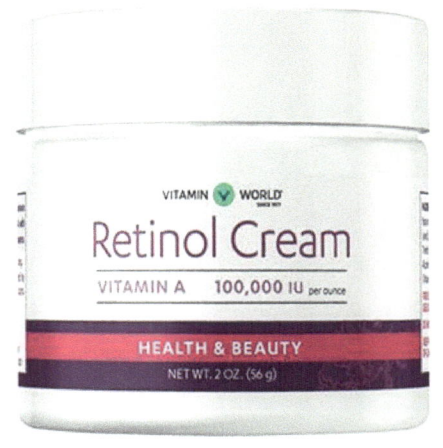

Most women use some sort of skin moisturizing product and these can be very costly. Retinol (or vitamin A cream) is one of the most effective products but can cost as much as $60 for only 4 oz! This formula contains 100,000IU of retinol per oz with a comparatively tiny price tag. Retinol has been shown to have remarkable anti-aging effects for the skin. This essential nutrient stimulates an increase in skin cells and activates others. Even 'aged' skin benefits from retinol cream.[4]

References

1.   Ballentine C. Biological differences may explain how women have survival advantage over men, new study finds. The Chronicle. https://www.dukechronicle.com/article/2018/01/biological-differences-may-explain-how-women-have-survival-advantage-over-men-new-study-finds. Published 2018. Accessed March 23, 2019.

2.   Angelo G, Drake V, Frei B. Efficacy of Multivitamin/mineral Supplementation to Reduce Chronic Disease Risk: A Critical Review of the Evidence from Observational Studies and Randomized Controlled Trials. Crit Rev Food Sci Nutr. 2014;55(14):1968-1991. doi:10.1080/10408398.2014.912199

3.   França K, Lotti T. *Advances In Integrative Dermatology*. Oxford: Wiley; :345-347.

4.   Shao Y, He T, Fisher G, Voorhees J, Quan T. Molecular basis of retinol anti-ageing properties in naturally aged human skinin vivo. *Int J Cosmet Sci*. 2016;39(1):56-65. doi:10.1111/ics.12348